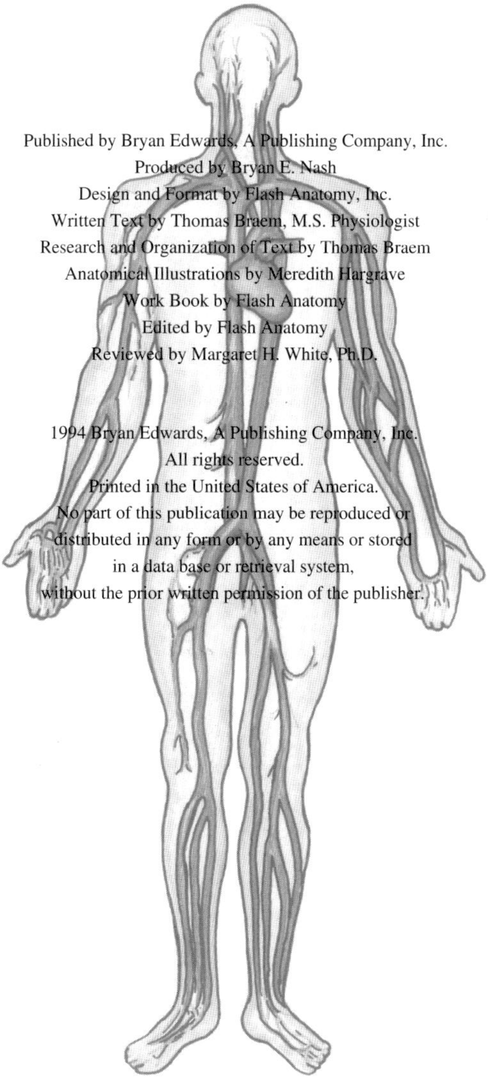

Published by Bryan Edwards, A Publishing Company, Inc.
Produced by Bryan E. Nash
Design and Format by Flash Anatomy, Inc.
Written Text by Thomas Braem, M.S. Physiologist
Research and Organization of Text by Thomas Braem
Anatomical Illustrations by Meredith Hargrave
Work Book by Flash Anatomy
Edited by Flash Anatomy
Reviewed by Margaret H. White, Ph.D.

Printed in the United States of America.

Printed on Recycled Paper

Nervous System

N_1

I. Nervous System Organization/Structures:

1. Nervous System Organization
   - A. Central (CNS) - Brain and Spinal Cord
   - B. Peripheral (PNS)
     1. Sensory
     2. Autonomic
        - a. Sympathetic
        - b. Parasympathetic
2. Nervous System Histology - Neurons
   - A. Structural Classification
     1. Unipolar, Bipolar, Multipolar
   - B. Functional Classification
     1. Sensory, Motor, Interneurons
3. Glial Cells
4. Impulse Transmission
   - A. Depolarization
   - B. Synapse/Neurotransmitters

II. CNS - Brain:

1. Brain (general views)
2. Brain Coverings
   - A. Cranium
   - B. Meninges
   - C. Cerebrospinal Fluid
3. Brainstem
   - A. Medulla
   - B. Pons
   - C. Midbrain
4. Diencephalon
   - A. Thalamus
   - B. Hypothalamus
5. Cerebrum
   - A. Cerebral Hemispheres
     1. Gray/White matter
   - B. Basal Nuclei
6. Limbic System
7. Cranial Nerves

III. CNS - Spinal Cord:

1. Spinal Cord
   - A. Longitudinal
   - B. Cross-section
2. Spinal Nerves
   - A. Plexus

IV. PNS - Divisions:

1. Sympathetic
2. Parasympathetic
3. Somatic
   - A. Neuromuscular junction

V. Reflex Arc:

1. Reflex Arc

Nervous System

N1

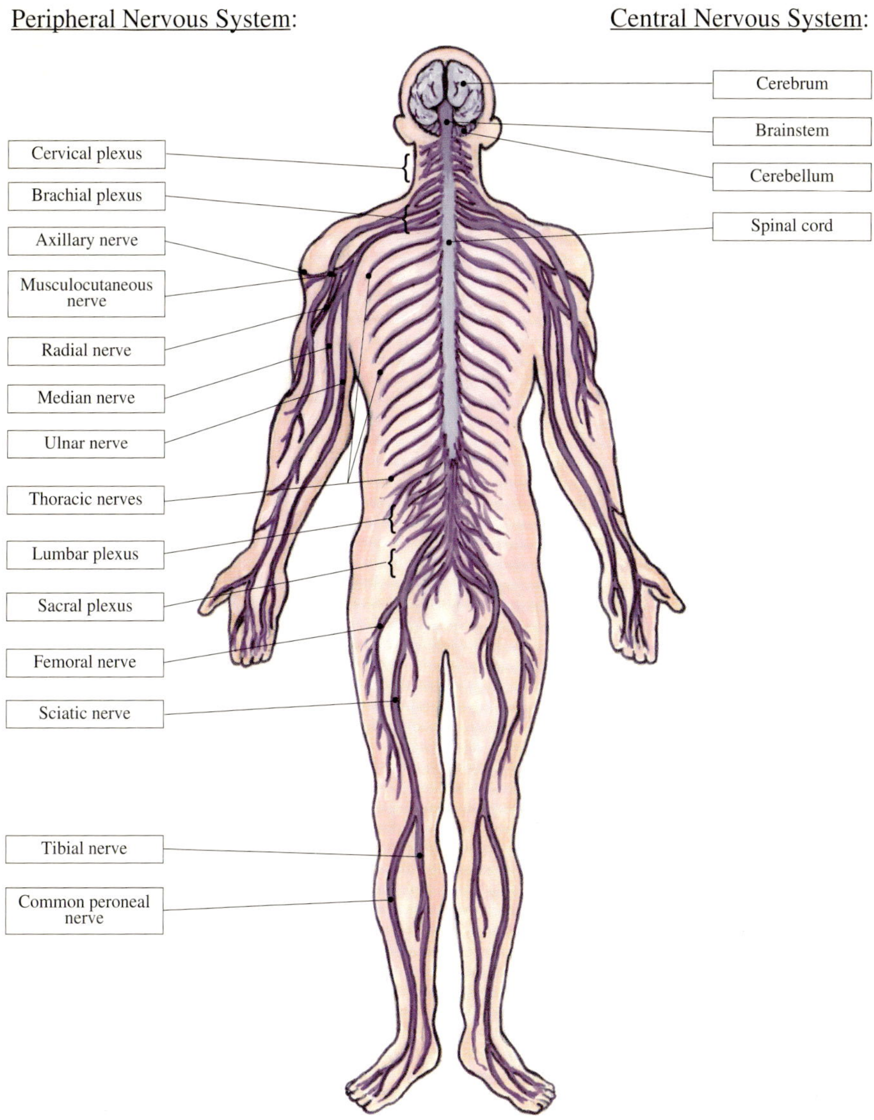

Anterior View

Neurons

N_2

I. Location:

1. Neurons are distributed throughout the brain and spinal cord, central nervous system (CNS), and throughout the tissues of the rest of the body, the peripheral nervous system (PNS)[1].

II. Structure:

1. Neurons typically consist of three distinct parts:
   A. Cell body: Contains the nucleus and organelles, surrounded by cytoplasm.
   B. Dendrites: Extensions from the cell body. There may be more than one dendrite per neuron.
   C. Axon: A single long process extending away from the body. Some axons have an insulating phospholipid coating, myelin[2], around them. Branches off the axon are called axon collaterals. Axons vary in length from a few millimeters to over a meter.

2. Neurons may be classified structurally based on the number of dendrites and axons:
   A. Unipolar neurons have one process from the cell body that then divides into branches that function as a dendrite and axon.
   B. Bipolar neurons have one dendrite and one axon projecting from the cell body.
   C. Multipolar neurons have several dendrites and one axon.

III. Function:

1. Neurons conduct nerve impulses. Specifically:
   A. Cell bodies contain the genetic material of the cell, and can regulate processes such as protein synthesis by organelles.
   B. Dendrites receive information from various receptors of the body or impulses from other neurons[2], and conduct impulses toward the cell body.
   C. Axons conduct impulses from the cell body to other neurons or cells of a target organ.

2. Neurons may be functionally classified according to the division of the nervous system to which they belong[1]:
   A. Sensory neurons conduct impulses toward the CNS.
   B. Motor neurons conduct impulses from the CNS.
   C. Association (interneurons) are located in the CNS and conduct impulses from sensory to motor neurons.

Cross-Reference

Volume	Chapter
1. N1	Nervous System
2. N4	Impulse Transmission

Definitions

Notes:

Neurons

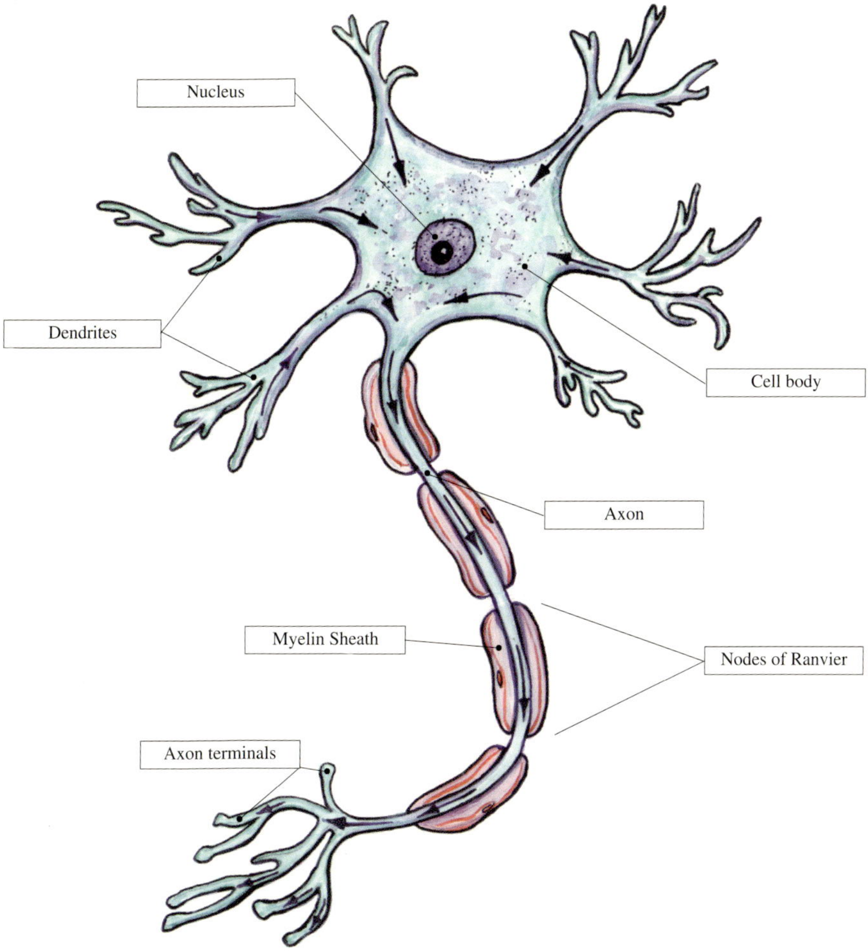

Multipolar Neuron

Glial Cells

N_3

I. Location:

1. Glial cells (neuroglia) are found throughout the nervous system[1].

2. Though glial cells make up the majority of the CNS[1] (90%), they tend to branch less extensively than neurons, and therefore make up about half of the volume of the CNS.

II. Structure:

1. Most glial cells are somewhat star-shaped, with a central cell body containing the nucleus and organelles, and varying numbers of processes projecting from the cell body.

2. Depending on shape and function, glial cells may be classified as astrocytes, oligodendrocytes, ependymal cells, or glial cells.

III. Function:

1. Glial cells generally support and protect the nervous system.

2. Astrocytes hold neurons together and attach neurons to structures such as blood vessels. They play a role in the repair of nervous tissue, and take up excess potassium from the fluid between the cells of the brain, preventing overexcitability.

3. Oligodendrocytes form supporting rows between neurons in the CNS, and form insulating myelin sheaths[2] around some axons in the CNS. Schwann cells form the sheaths around myelinated axons of the PNS.

4. Ependymal cells line cavities in the CNS such as the ventricles of the brain and central canal of the spinal cord. They contribute to the formation of cerebrospinal fluid[3].

5. Microglia are phagocytic cells from the blood that scavenge and engulf debris. Generally stationary, they may become activated and migrate to the site of injury or infection.

Cross-Reference

Volume	Chapter
1. N1	Nervous System
2. N4	Impulse Transmission
3. N7	Brain Coverings

Definitions

Notes:

Glial Cells

Astocytes

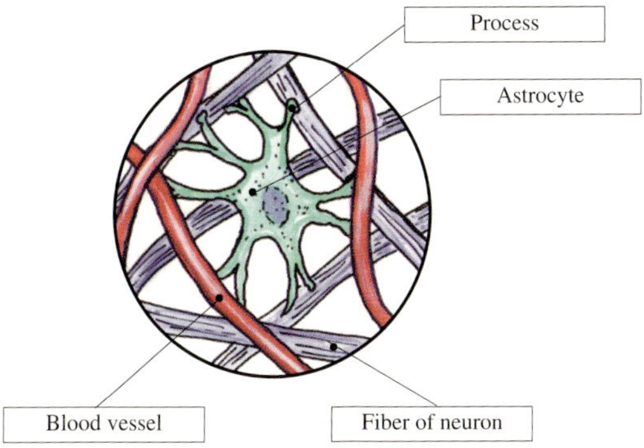

Oligodendrocytes

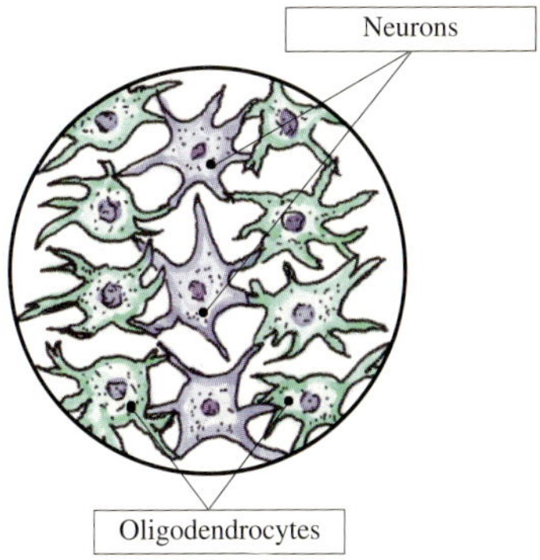

Microglia

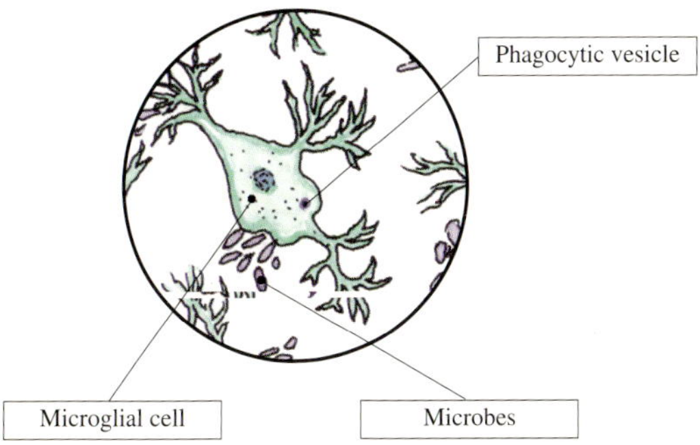

Ependymal

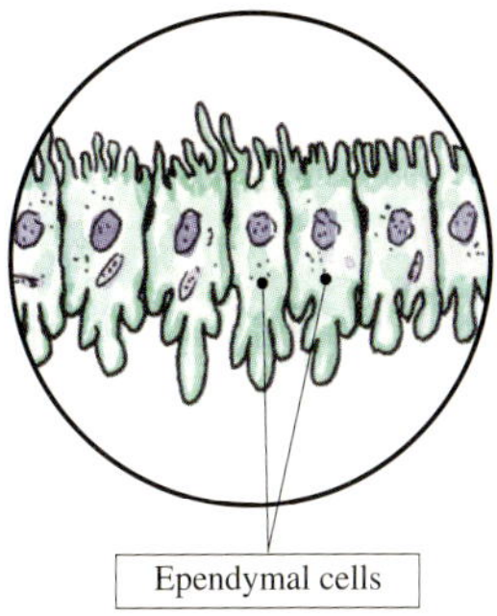

Microscopic views

Impulse Transmission

N_4

I. Location:

1. Transmission of impulses takes place throughout the nervous system[1].

II. Structure:

1. In a resting neuron, there exists an unequal distribution of ions on either side of the plasma membrane of the neuron.

2. This unequal distribution creates a net charge difference between the inside and outside of the plasma membrane (membrane potential, resting potential). Such a membrane is said to be polarized.

III. Function:

1. The unequal distribution of charges is due to:
   A. Large negatively-charged ions that are trapped inside the cell that cannot diffuse out.
   B. The functioning of sodium pumps that actively transport these ions out of the cell, and potassium pumps that transport these ions in to the cell.

2. Upon proper stimulation, the permeability of the membrane to sodium is greatly increased, and sodium ions flood into the cell. The net charge on the sides of the plasma membrane quickly reverses, and the membrane becomes depolarized.

3. This depolarization, or wave of charge reversal, is what constitutes a nerve impulse or action potential.

4. Resting potential is quickly restored as potassium diffuses through the more permeable membrane to the outside of the cell. This process is called repolarization. The pumps then restore the ions to their resting positions.

5. A brief period exists while repolarization occurs, known as the refractory period, during which time another depolarization may not occur. The refractory period prevents the impulse from traveling back toward its point of origin. Therefore, neurons may only conduct impulses in one direction.

6. In myelinated axons[2], depolarization need only occur in the area of the axon exposed between the insulating myelin sheath. This "jumping" of the action potential from gap to gap is known as saltatory transmission. Transmission through myelinated axons is therefore much faster than in unmyelinated axons.

Cross-Reference

Volume	Chapter
1. N1	Nervous System
2. N19	Somatic Nervous System

Definitions

1. Ion: A charged particle.

Notes:

Impulse Transmission

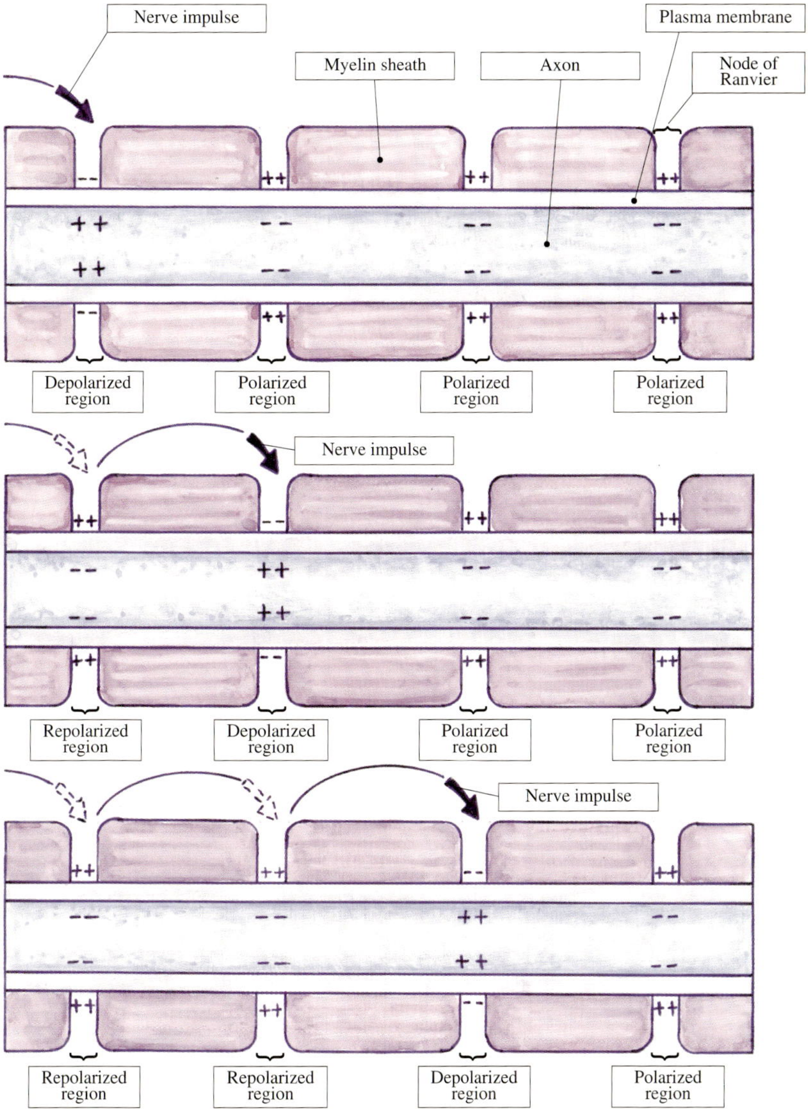

Synaptic Transmission

N_5

I. Location:

1. Synaptic transmission occurs throughout the nervous system[1].

II. Structure:

1. Neurons do not come into physical contact with each other, but are separated by gaps known as synapses. The neuron before the synapse may be called presynaptic, and the neuron after the synapse called postsynaptic.

2. Gaps exist between neurons and cells that are the target of their impulses as well. An example is that of a neuromuscular junction[2].

3. Chemicals known as neurotransmitters are stored in sacs in the ends of axons (axon terminals)[3]. Common neurotransmitters include acetylcholine, norepinephrine, dopamine, and serotonin.

III. Function:

1. Upon propagation to the end of an axon terminal, an action potential[4] triggers the opening of calcium channels in the end of the axon terminal in the presynaptic neuron.

2. Calcium stimulates the release of the neurotransmitter from the presynaptic neuron.

3. Neurotransmitters bind to specific sites on the postsynaptic neuron, and alter its permeability to the ions that initiate an action potential.

4. The effect of the neurotransmitter on the postsynaptic neuron may be either excitatory or inhibitory. Excitatory effects make the postsynaptic neuron move closer to depolarization. Inhibitory effects make the postsynaptic neuron more polarized.

5. Most postsynaptic neurons receive input from many presynaptic neurons. The initiation of an action potential in a postsynaptic neuron depends on the sum of all the excitatory and inhibitory input from presynaptic neurons.

6. In this manner, neurotransmitters transmit or prevent the transmission of nerve impulses from one neuron to another, or from a neuron to its target cell.

Cross-Reference

Volume	Chapter
1. N1	Nervous System
2. N19	Somatic Nervous System
3. N2	Neurons
4. N4	Impulse Transmission

Definitions

Notes:

Synaptic Transmission

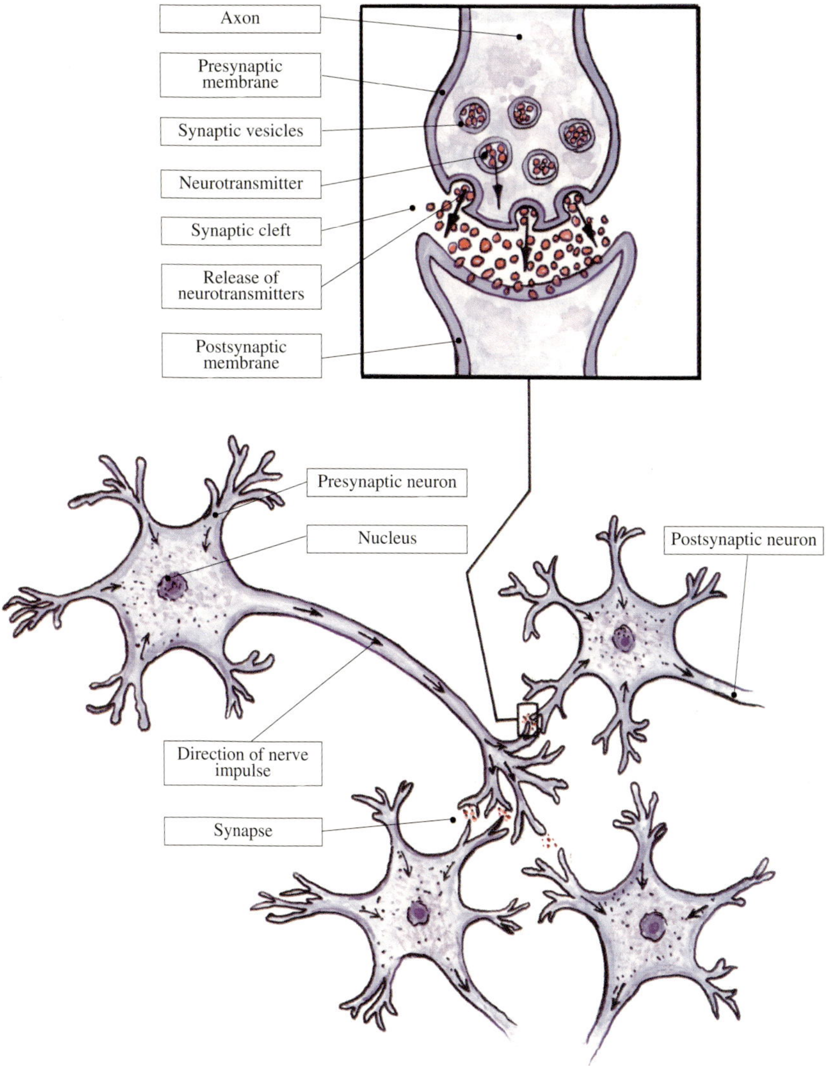

Brain

N6

I. Location:

1. The brain is enclosed by the cranial bones and meninges[1].

2. The lower brain continues down as the upper spinal cord.

II. Structure:

1. The brain is composed of nervous tissue - neurons, and glial cells.

2. The average adult brain weighs approximately 1300 grams.

3. The brain consists of four major parts:
   A. The cerebrum, which constitutes about 80% of the brain weight, includes the basal nuclei and cerebral cortex.
   B. The diencephalon, consisting of the thalamus and hypothalamus. The diencephalon and cerebrum together make up the forebrain.
   C. The brain stem, consisting of the medulla, pons, and midbrain.
   D. The cerebellum lies posterior to the brain stem and inferior to the cerebrum.

III. Function:

1. The brain processes input from the peripheral nervous system and spinal cord.

2. The brain directs the activities of the organs of the body.

3. The brain works in concert with the endocrine system[2] to control and coordinate the activities of the body.

4. The brain is responsible for complex intellectual and individual phenomena such as personality, thought, memory, language, and self-awareness.

Cross-Reference

Volume	Chapter
1. N7	Brain Coverings
2. E1	Endocrine System

Definitions

Notes:

Brain

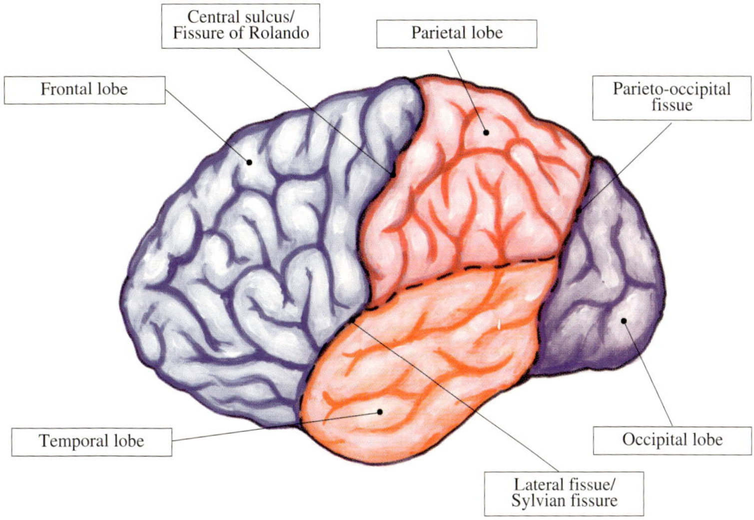

Lateral view

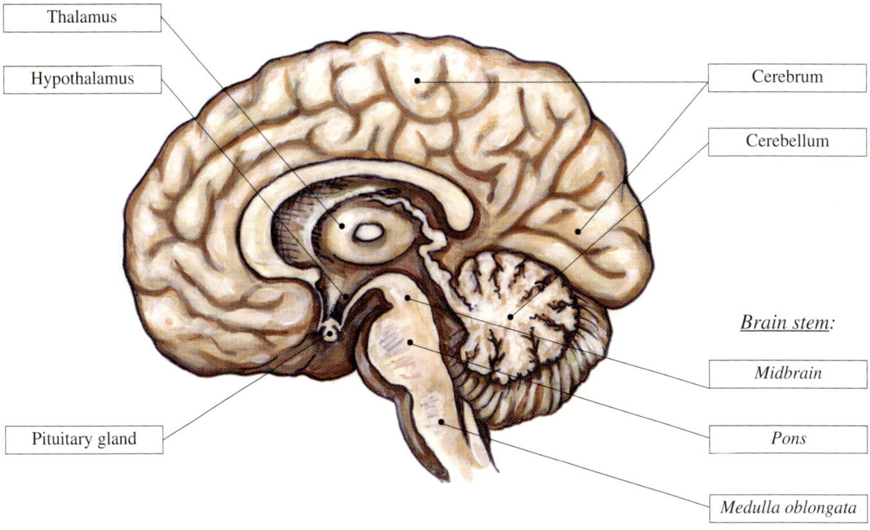

Sagittal view

Brain Coverings

N_7

I. Location:

1. The brain is protected by the cranial bones: the frontal, occipital, parietals, temporals, sphenoid, and ethmoid.
2. The meninges are coverings that surround both the brain and the spinal cord.
3. Cerebrospinal fluid fills cavities in the brain known as ventricles[1], the space between the arachnoid and pia mater (subarachnoid space) around the brain and spinal cord, and the central canal of the spinal cord[2].

II. Structure:

1. The outer meninx, the dura mater, is made of fibrous connective tissue. Around the brain it has two layers, with the outer layer attaching to the surrounding cranial bones. The inner layer alone continues down around the spinal cord.
2. The middle meninx, the arachnoid, is a delicate connective tissue layer. Between the dura mater and arachnoid is the subdural space containing a serous fluid.
3. The inner meninx, the pia mater, is a clear fibrous membrane that adheres to the outer surface of the brain and spinal cord. The subarachnoid space exists between the arachnoid and the pia mater, and is filled with cerebrospinal fluid.
4. Cerebrospinal fluid consists of water, proteins, glucose, salts, white blood cells, and urea. There is approximately 125ml. of cerebrospinal fluid surrounding the brain and spinal cord. It is formed in the ventricles of the brain.

III. Function:

1. The cranium serves as bony protection for the brain.
2. The meninges protect the brain as well. The subdural space acts as a fluid-filled cushion around the brain.
3. Cerebrospinal fluid absorbs shock and circulates nutrients from the blood to the brain tissues. The white blood cells may help in defense against inflammation and infection.
4. Exchange between the capillaries feeding the brain and the CSF is highly selective. This blood-brain barrier protects the brain tissue from many fluctuations of substances in the blood which could be harmful to delicate brain tissue.

Cross-Reference

Volume	Chapter
1. N8	Ventricles
2. N16	Spinal Cord

Definitions

Notes:

Brain Coverings

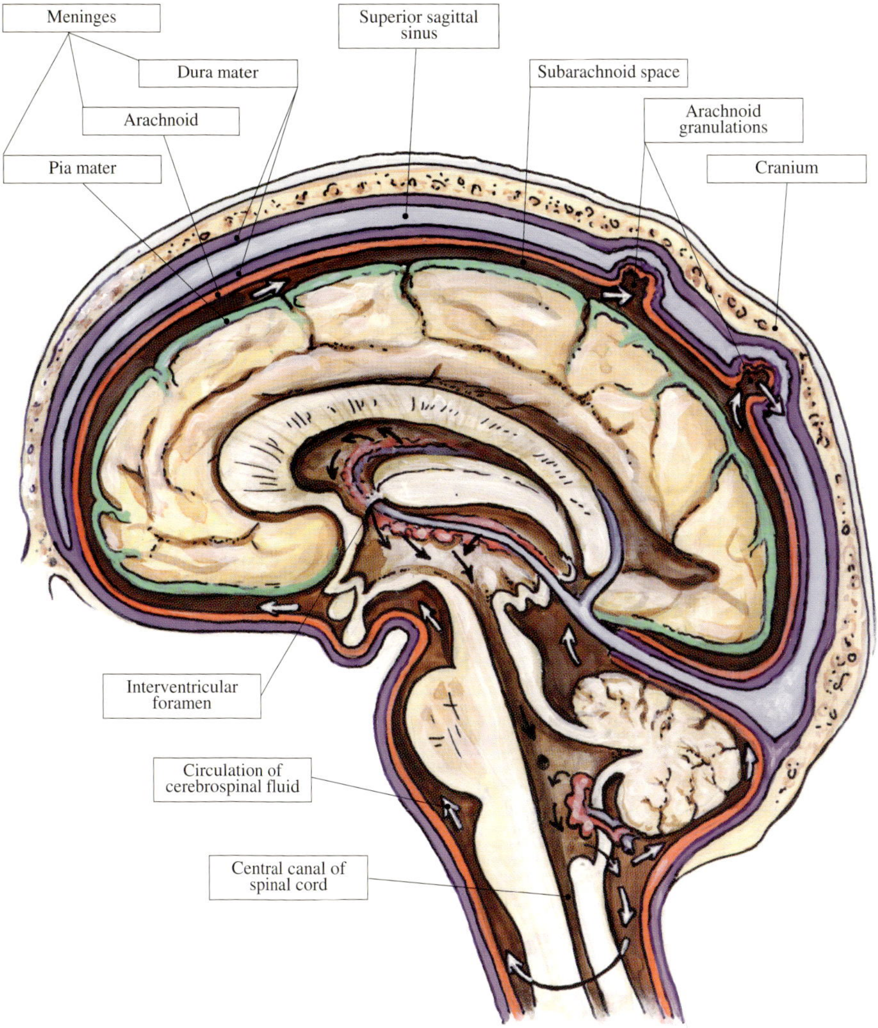

Left lateral view

Ventricles

N_8

I. Location:

1. The ventricles are cavities located within the brain.

2. Each of the two lateral ventricles is located in a cerebral hemisphere[1].

3. The third ventricle is a thin slit between the lateral ventricles and the left and right halves of the thalamus.

4. The third ventricle is connected to each lateral ventricle by a small opening, the interventricular foramen (foramen of Monro).

5. The fourth ventricle is located between the cerebellum and the lower brain stem.

6. The third and fourth ventricles are connected by a small canal, the cerebral aqueduct (aqueduct of Sylvius). The fourth ventricle also opens to the subarachnoid space between the inner meninges[2] by a median and two lateral apertures, and to the central canal of the spinal cord.

II. Structure:

1. The ventricles are cavities within the brain tissue.

2. The ventricles are lined by ependymal cells, a type of glial cell[3].

3. Ependymal cells and capillaries from the inner meninx and pia mater, form a network called the choroid plexus.

III. Function:

1. The choroid plexuses from each ventricle secrete cerebrospinal fluid[2].

2. Cerebrospinal fluid flows from the lateral ventricles to the third ventricle via the interventricular foramen. The third ventricle contributes more fluid, which flows to the fourth ventricle via the cerebral aqueduct. The fourth ventricle adds more fluid, which then can flow through the apertures from the fourth ventricle to the subarachnoid space around the brain and spinal cord.

Cross-Reference

Volume	Chapter
1. N12	Cerebrum
2. N7	Brain Coverings
3. N3	Glial Cells

Definitions

Notes:

Ventricles

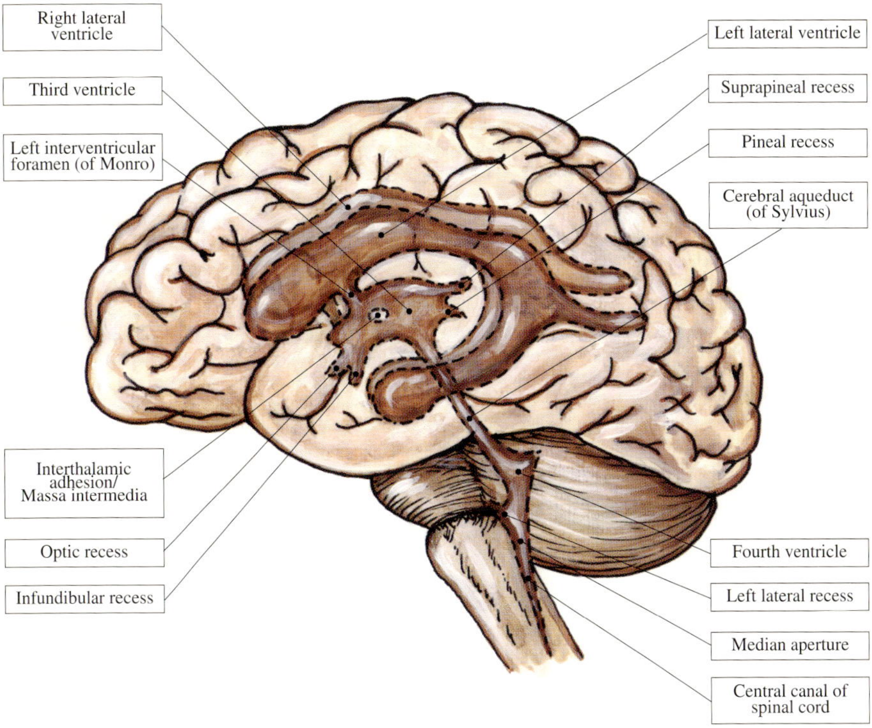

Left lateral view

Brain Stem

N9

I. Location:

1. The brain stem is the lowest portion of the brain and is continuous with the spinal cord. It consists of three basic parts: the medulla, the pons, and the midbrain[1].

II. Structure:

1. The medulla oblongata or medulla, is a continuation of the spinal cord and measures approximately 3cm. in length.

2. The pons varolii or pons, is situated directly above the medulla and in front of the cerebellum. It is approximately 2.5cm. long.

3. The midbrain lies directly above the pons and below the diencephalon[2]. It measures about 2.5cm. in length.

III. Function:

1. The brain stem serves as a pathway for all ascending and descending input between the spinal cord and higher brain centers. The brain stem also functions in the regulation of many vegetative functions of the body.

2. The medulla helps regulate many vital functions of the body, such as heart beat, blood vessel diameter, breathing, digestive functioning, consciousness, and arousal.

3. The pons' roles are primarily concerned with acting as a bridge between the spinal cord and brain, and between brain parts. Contributions to control of respiration, sleep, and other activities come from the pons as well.

4. The midbrain serves as a connection to upper brain structures, as well as regulating many eye and head reflexes to different stimuli.

5. Many cranial nerves[3] arise from various portions of the brain stem.

Cross-Reference

Volume	Chapter
1. N6	Brain
2. N11	Diencephalon
3. N15	Cranial Nerves

Definitions

Notes:

Brain Stem

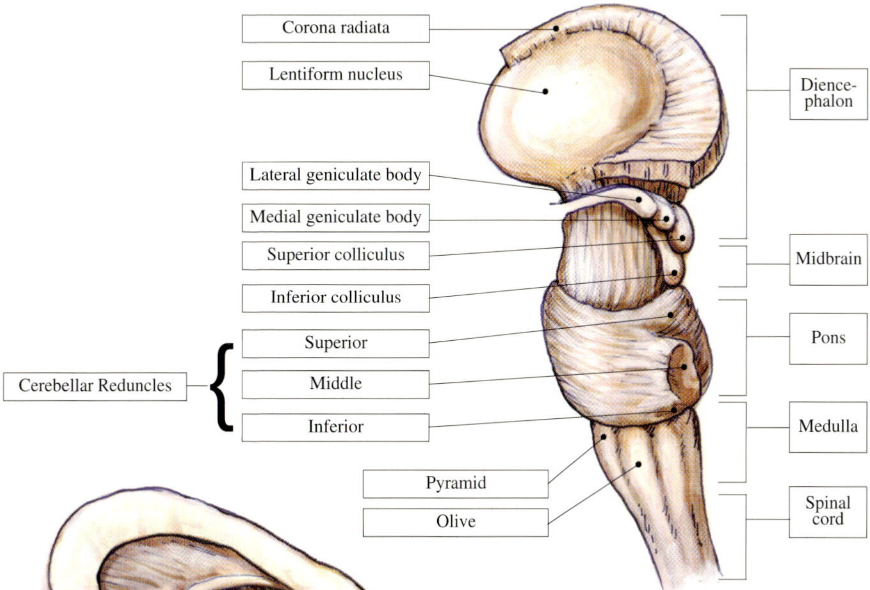

Lateral view

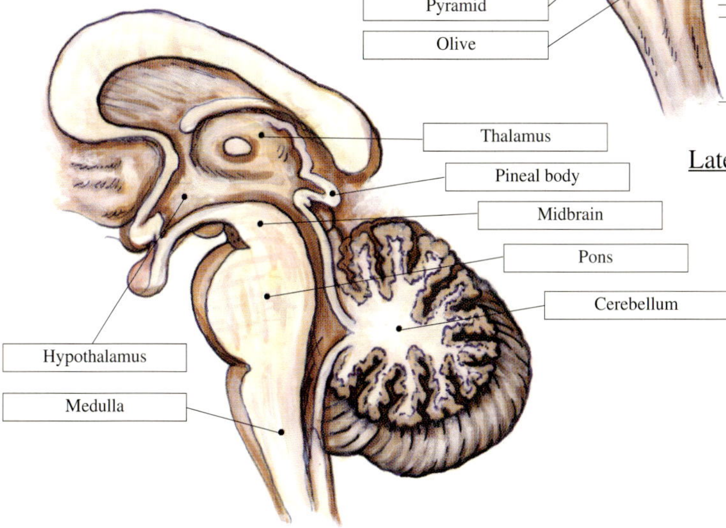

Median sagittal view

Cerebellum

N_{10}

I. Location:

1. The cerebellum is located posterior to the brain stem and inferior to the occipital lobe of the cerebral cortex[1].

II. Structure:

1. The cerebellum is divided into a central vermis and lateral hemispheres.

2. Bundles of fibers known as peduncles connect the cerebellum to the brain stem.

3. The cerebellum consists of an outer layer of gray matter around an inner white core[2].

4. The surface of the cerebellum is corrugated by slender ridges known as folia or gyri.

III. Function:

1. The cerebellum, with input from many other parts of the nervous system, maintains proper balance and posture.

2. Maintenance of muscle tone occurs in the cerebellum.

3. The cerebellum has large roles in the coordination of sequential and repetitive movements.

Cross-Reference

Volume	Chapter
1. N6	Brain
2. N12	Cerebrum

Definitions

Notes:

Cerebellum

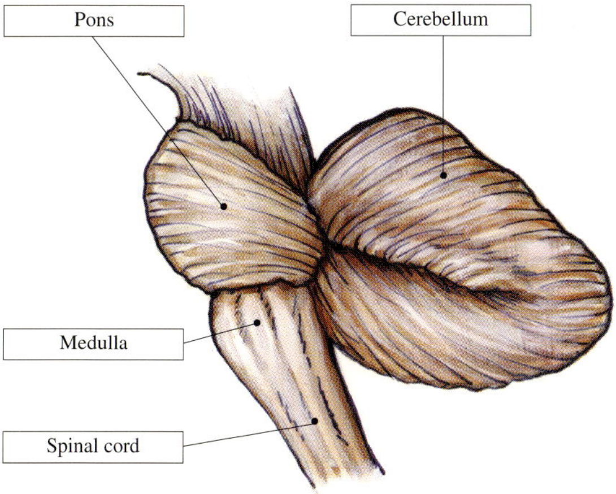

Left lateral view

Vermis of Cerebellum:

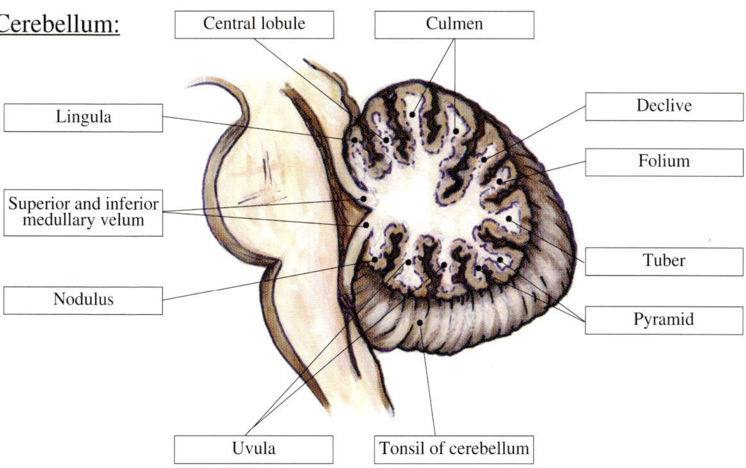

Sagittal view

Diencephalon

N_{11}

I. Location:

1. The diencephalon lies anterior to the midbrain and inferior to the cerebrum[1].

II. Structure:

1. The diencephalon is separated into two lateral halves by the third ventricle[2]. The two halves are joined in most human brains.

2. Each half can be divided into a thalamus and hypothalamus.

3. The thalamus is the posterior portion of the diencephalon, consists of gray matter surrounded by a thin layer of white matter, and is approximately 3cm. long.

4. The hypothalamus is a very small collection of primarily gray matter anterior and inferior to the thalamus. A stalk, the infundibulum, extends down from the hypothalamus and connects it to the pituitary gland[3].

III. Function:

1. The thalamus serves as the principal relay station for input from the periphery and other brain parts to the cerebral cortex.

2. The thalamus screens some input, participates in a basic level of awareness and consciousness, and motor control.

3. The hypothalamus is the regulating center for many homeostatic functions such as temperature, thirst, hunger, and satiety.

4. Specialized neurons in the hypothalamus produce the hormones vasopressin and oxytocin, and secrete them into the blood through the posterior pituitary. Vasopressin stimulates water retention by the kidneys, while oxytocin produces uterine contraction and milk ejection.

5. The hypothalamus stimulates release of many hormones from the anterior pituitary through connections in the infundibulum. The connections between the hypothalamus and pituitary gland provide the major link between the nervous and endocrine systems.

6. The hypothalamus plays a role in emotions and many basic behavioral patterns.

Cross-Reference

Volume	Chapter
1. N6	Brain
2. N7	Brain Covereings
3. E5	Pituitary Gland

Definitions

1. Homeostatic: Concerned with maintenance of internal conditions of the body in ranges ideal for survival.

Notes:

Diencephalon

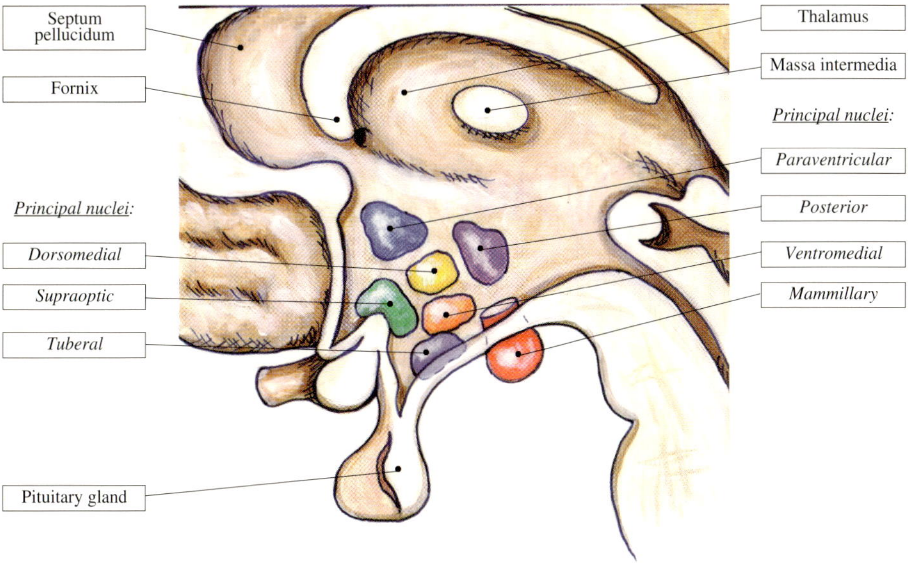

Hypothalamus: Median sagittal section

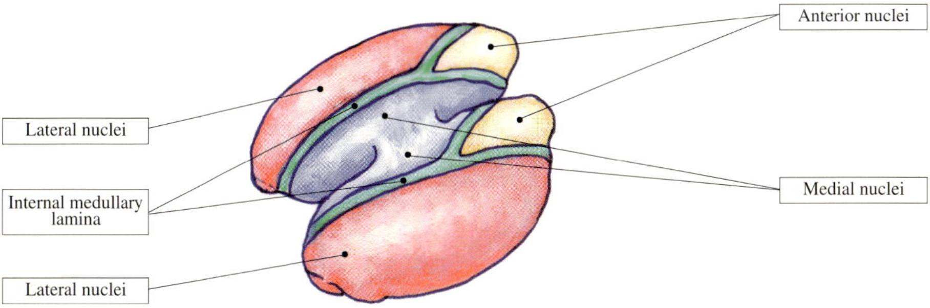

Thalamus superior/lateral view

Cerebrum

N_{12}

I. Location:

1. The cerebrum constitutes the bulk of the brain. It lies above the brain stem, diencephalon, and cerebellum[1].

II. Structure:

1. The cerebrum is composed of an outer layer of gray matter approximately 1.3 - 4.5mm. thick, called the cerebral cortex.
2. The gray matter is highly folded into gyri (convolutions) separated by fissures or sulci.
3. The longitudinal fissure separates the cortex into a left and right hemisphere.
4. Each hemisphere is divided by deep fissures (sulci) into four lobes named for the protective cranial bones over them:
   A. The central sulcus separates the frontal and parietal lobes.
   B. The lateral fissure separates the frontal and temporal lobes.
   C. The parieto-occipital fissures separates the parietal and occipital lobes.
5. Underneath the thin gray matter cortex lies the white matter which composes the majority of the cerebrum. Grey matter is composed primarily of cell bodies and dendrites, whereas white matter is basically myelinated axons[2].
6. Deep within the white matter of the cerebrum and lateral to the thalamus[3] lies a mass of gray matter called the basal nuclei.

III. Function:

1. The cerebral cortex functions in most higher thought processes. Though no portion of the brain seems to work totally independently of other areas, some regional specialization does exist. Chapter N13 lists many of these functional areas.
2. The left hemisphere generally excels at thought processes needing fragmentary analysis such as math, sequential problems, logical thought, and the use of language.
3. The right hemisphere specializes in holistic or creative thought processes such as music, art, or spatial perception.
4. The basal nuclei relies on its many connections to the thalamus, cerebral cortex, and brain stem to accomplish its functions. These include roles in selecting useful and inhibiting useless movements, the regulation of muscle tone, and coordination of other slow, sustained contractions of muscles.

Cross-Reference

Volume	Chapter
1. N6	Brain
2. N2	Neurons
3. N11	Diencephalon

Definitions

Notes:

Cerebrum

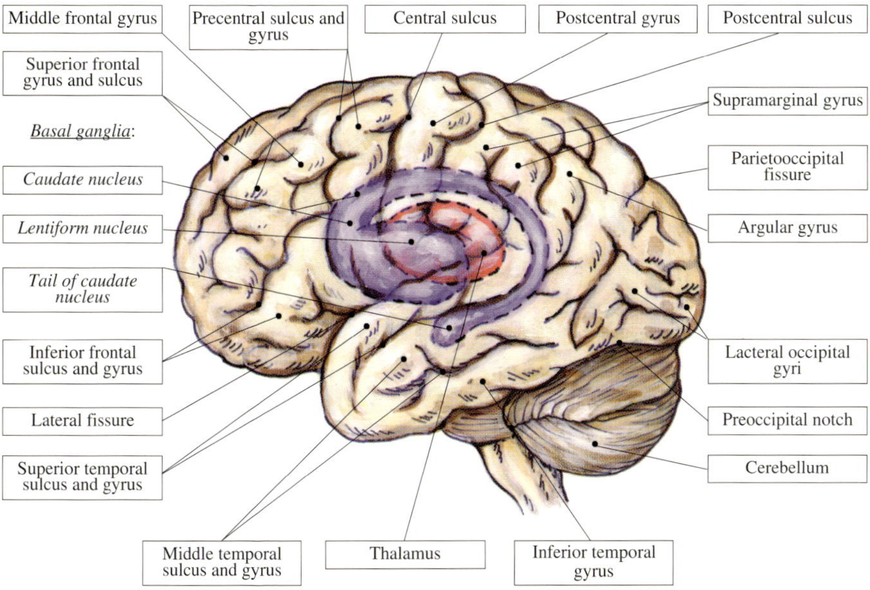

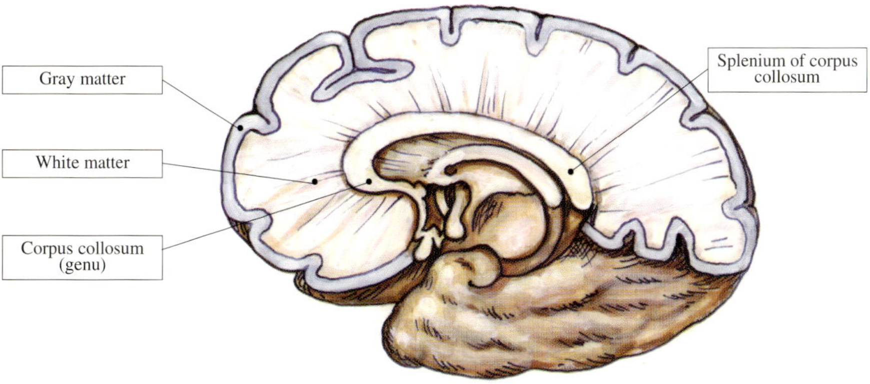

Median sagittal view

Functional Areas - Cerebral Cortex

N_{13}

I. Location:

1. See Volume N10, Cerebrum.

II. Structure:

1. Parts of the cerebral cortex do not function independently of other portions of the nervous system. Each receives input from many other parts of the cortex or other areas of the brain. This being understood, different areas do play key roles in certain cerebral activities.

III. Function:

1. The frontal lobes of the cerebral cortex function in conversion of thought to speech, ability to speak, and voluntary motor control. The primary motor cortex lies at the posterior edge of this lobe, and controls voluntary skeletal muscle movements.

2. The parietal lobes process sensory input from the skin and related structures, as well as perception of the position of body in space. The area that processes this input is a region just behind the central sulcus known as the somatosensory cortex.

3. The temporal lobes receive and process information about sound sensation.

4. Initial processing of visual input occurs in the occipital lobe.

5. Wernicke's area, a region of both the parietal and temporal lobes of the left hemisphere, functions in the comprehension of verbal and written language.

6. In the left frontal lobe, Broca's area plays a key role in the ability to speak.

7. Association areas consist of portions of most of the cerebral cortex. These areas are responsible for processes, such as complex motor control, sensation, personality, reasoning, and most complex cognitive functions.

Cross-Reference
Volume Chapter

Definitions

Notes:

Functional Areas - Cerebral Cortex

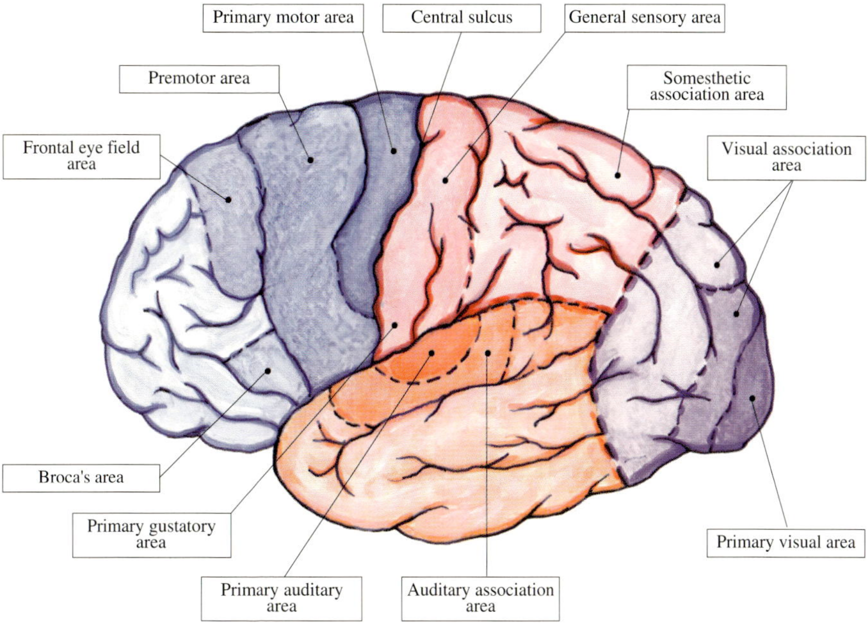

= Frontal lobe
= Parietal lobe
= Temporal lobe
= Occipitial lobe

Limbic System

N_{14}

I. Location:

1. The limbic system is not a separate structure in the brain, but consists of portions of several other brain parts, including the cerebral cortex, basal nuclei of the cerebrum, and portions of the diencephalon[1].

II. Structure:

1. The limbic system is basically an association of gray matter from several higher brain structures[2]. Areas of the limbic system, including the amygdala, hippocampus, cingulate gyrus, mammillary body, and fornix are seen on the facing illustration.

III. Function:

1. The limbic system plays key roles in emotional behavior and emotional responses to various stimuli.

2. The limbic system functions in learning and memory.

3. Sociosexual behavior, such as sexual drives, is greatly influenced by the limbic system.

4. In many animals, this area has direct connections with the smell and olfactory areas of the brain. These links suggest roles for the limbic system in the integration of hormonal and glandular secretions and mating drives/seasons. The significance of this integration in humans is unclear.

Cross-Reference

Volume	Chapter
1. N6	Brain
2. N12	Cerebrum

Definitions

Notes:

Limbic System

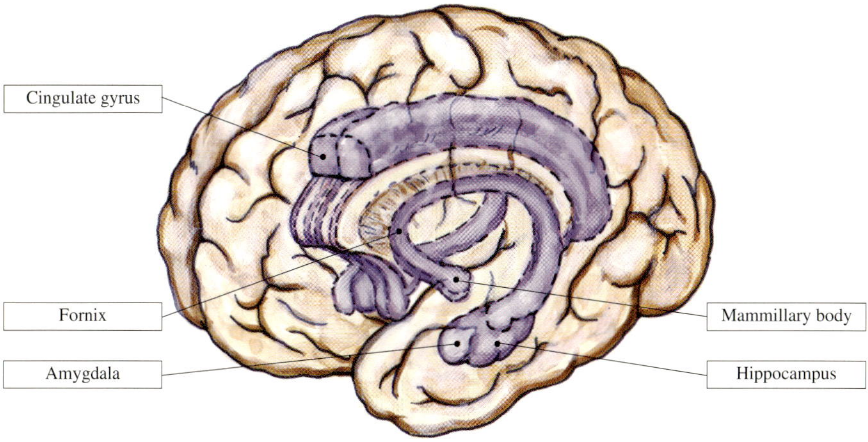

Lateral view turned slightly to the left

Fornix

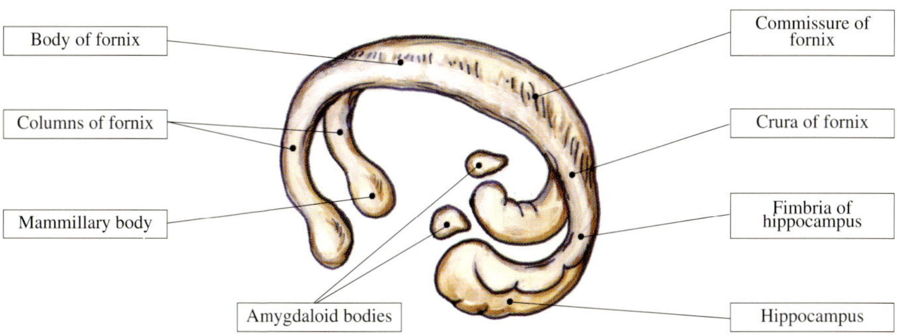

Left lateral view

Cranial Nerves

N_{15}

I. Location:

1. The cranial nerves originate in the brain stem, upper brain or spinal cord, and communicate with various parts of the body.

2. Cranial nerves are paired nerves, one on each side of the brain.

3. Cranial nerves may be numbered by a Roman numeral indicating the order of their appearance from the brain (front to back), or by a name corresponding to their function (see illustration).

II. Structure:

1. The cranial nerves consist of neurons and their associated glial cells.

2. Some cranial nerves consist of sensory neurons only, whereas some contain both sensory and motor fibers (mixed).

III. Function:

1. Cranial nerves convey information to/from the brain. Some of the specific roles of individual cranial nerves are:

   I. Sensory: Input on smell from the nose to cerebral cortex.
   II. Sensory: Vision input from eye to the thalamus.
   III. Mixed: Muscles of the eye and pupil to/from the midbrain.
   IV. Mixed: Muscles of the eyeball to/from the midbrain.
   V. Mixed: Face and scalp to the pons, pons to muscles of chewing.
   VI. Mixed: Muscles of the eyeball to/from the pons.
   VII. Mixed: Taste buds and skin of ear to the pons. Pons muscles of facial expression.
   VIII. Sensory: Hearing and equilibrium input from inner ear to the thalamus and cerebellum.
   IX. Mixed: Taste buds and carotid sinus to the thalamus. Medulla to some salivary glands and muscles of swallowing.
   X. Mixed: Visceral organs such as heart, lungs, and digestive organs to the medulla/pons. Medulla to many visceral organs.
   XI. Mixed: Muscles of the throat and anterior neck to/from the medulla and cervical portion of the spinal cord.
   XII. Mixed. Muscles of the tongue to/from the medulla.

Cross-Reference **Definitions**

Volume Chapter

Notes:

Cranial Nerves

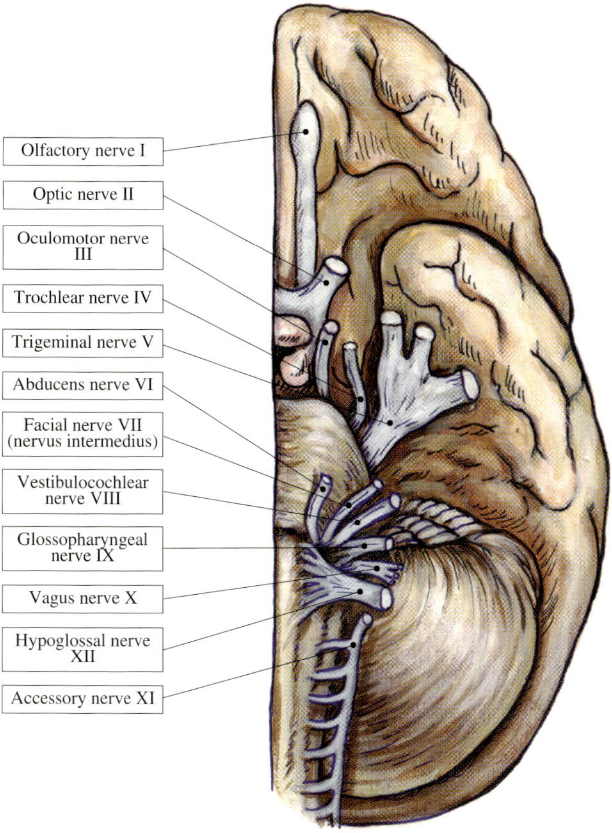

Inferior view / left cerebrum

Spinal Cord

N_{16}

I. Location:

1. The spinal cord in enclosed in the vertebral column, and runs from the lower brain stem at the foramen magnum of the occipital bone to the level of the second lumbar vertebra.

II. Structure:

1. The spinal cord is an oval-shaped cylinder less than an inch in diameter and approximately 42 to 45cm. in length.

2. In cross-section, the spinal cord can be seen to consists of a central butterfly-shaped mass of gray matter surrounded by white matter.

3. The gray matter consists primarily of neuron cell bodies, dendrites, unmyelinated axons, or glial cells.

4. White matter consists primarily of myelinated axons. These fibers run vertically in columns known as tracts.

5. The spinal cord is surrounded by meninges, cerebrospinal fluid, adipose tissue, and blood vessels[1].

6. Paired spinal nerves arise from the spinal cord[2]. Each spinal nerve communicates with the spinal cord by two short roots.

7. The anterior (ventral) root contains motor fibers, whereas the posterior (dorsal) root contains sensory fibers. The roots unite into a mixed spinal nerve shortly beyond the spinal cord[2].

III. Function:

1. The spinal cord is a pathway for neurons to and from the brain and peripheral nervous tissues or target organs.

2. Ascending tracts convey impulses from the periphery to the brain, while descending tracts carry motor impulses from the brain to peripheral targets.

3. The spinal cord integrates input from peripheral sensory neurons and may initiate reflex motor impulses to be carried to an effector[3].

Cross-Reference

Volume	Chapter
1. N7	Brain Coverings
2. N17	Spinal Nerves
3. N20	Reflex Arc

Definitions

Notes:

Spinal Cord

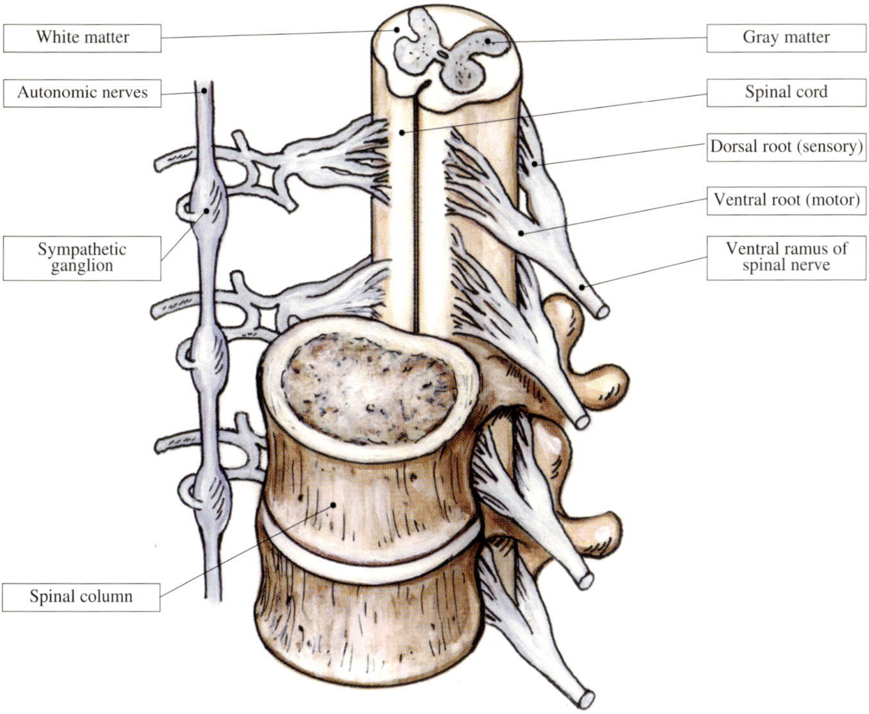

Anterior view rotated slightly to the right

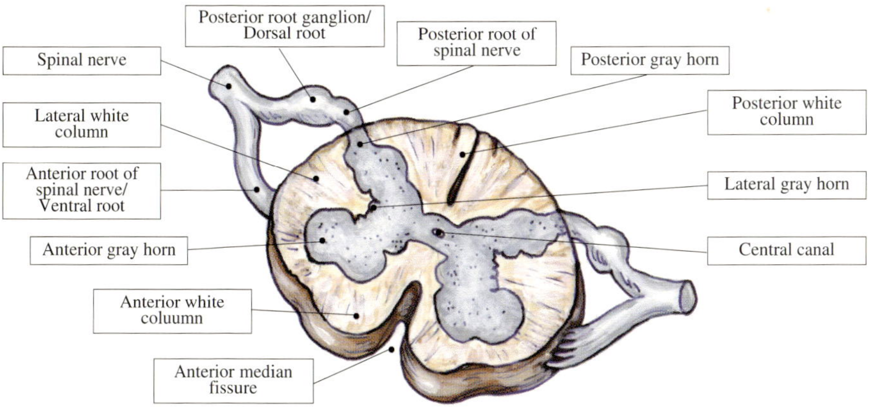

Cross-section

Spinal Nerves

N_{17}

I. Location:

1. The 31 pairs of spinal nerves arise from the spinal cord.
2. The first pair emerges between the occipital bone and the first cervical vertebra. The other pairs of spinal nerves emerge from the intervertebral foramina between adjacent vertebrae. Since the spinal cord ends at about L2, nerves below this point continue as the cauda equina before emerging from the spine.
3. Named for the vertebra above which they emerge, there are 8 cervical, 12 thoracic, 5 lumbar, 5 sacral, and 1 coccygeal pair of spinal nerves.

II. Structure:

1. Each mixed spinal nerve attaches to the spinal cord via two short roots, one anterior and one posterior[1].
2. Each individual fiber in the spinal nerve is covered and bundled together into a spinal nerve by connective tissue wrappings, the endoneurium, perineurium, and epineurium. The epineurium is continuous with the meninges[2].
3. Each spinal nerve branches into rami shortly after leaving the spinal cord. The rami communicantes (white rami) contain fibers of the autonomic nervous system[3]. The posterior rami supply the muscles and skin of the posterior head, neck, and trunk. Anterior (ventral) rami of all spinal nerves, except T2-T12, form interbranching networks called plexuses shortly after leaving the spinal cord. There is no thoracic plexus.

III. Function:

1. Spinal nerves carry information to and from the spinal cord and the periphery.
2. The cervical plexus supplies the skin and muscles of the head, neck, upper shoulders, and diaphragm.
3. The brachial plexus supplies the upper extremities, neck, and shoulder regions.
4. Thoracic spinal nerves T2-T12 supply the skin and muscles of the chest, abdomen, and back.
5. The lumbar plexus supplies some of the lower extremity, external genitals, and abdominal wall.
6. The sacral plexus supplies the lower extremities and buttocks.

Cross-Reference

Volume	Chapter
1. N16	Spinal Cord
2. N7	Brain Coverings
3. N18	Autonomic Nervous System

Definitions

Notes:

Spinal Nerves

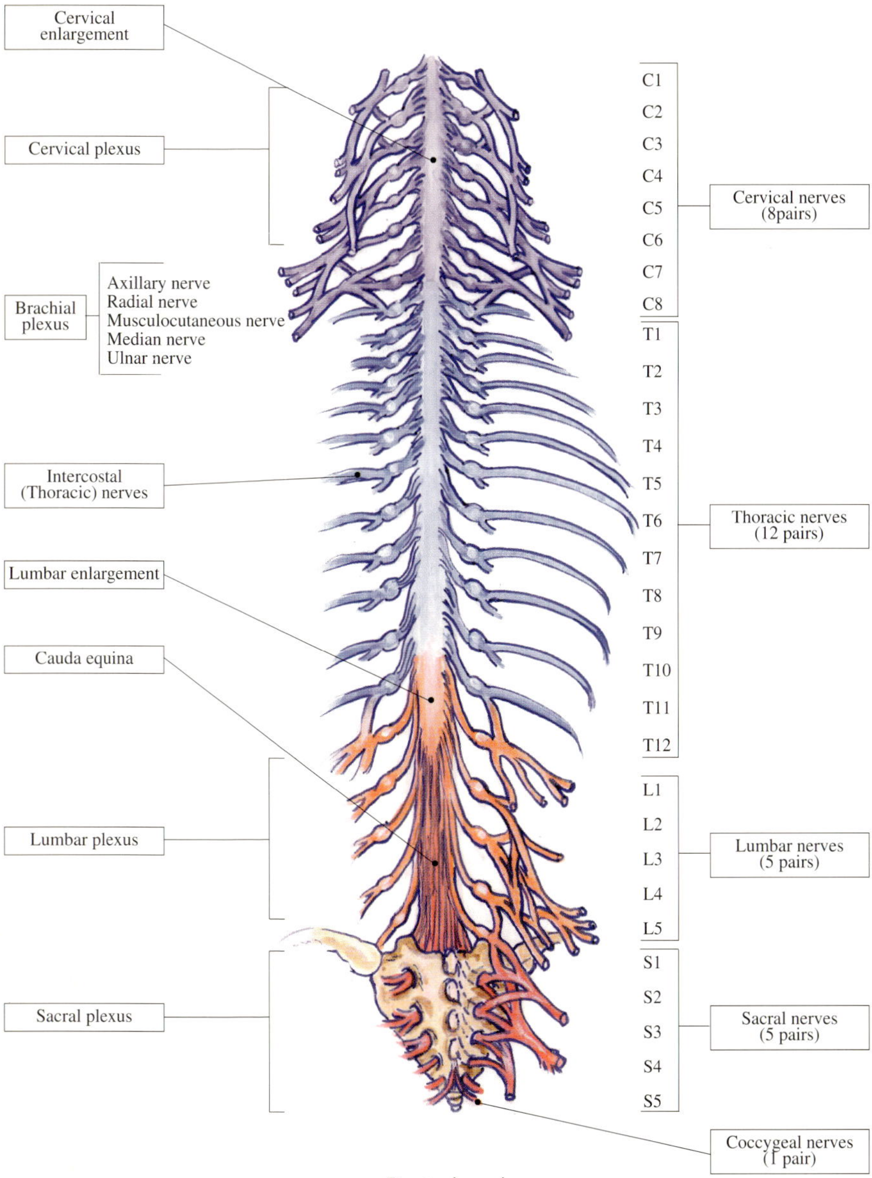

Posterior view

Autonomic Nervous System (Part I)

N_{18A}

I. Location:

1. The autonomic nervous system (ANS) is not a separate system, but a division of the nervous system consisting of motor neurons that innervate smooth muscle, cardiac muscle, and glands[1].

2. Many organs innervated by the ANS receive input from two distinct branches of the ANS, the sympathetic and parasympathetic divisions. These organs therefore exhibit dual innervation.

II. Structure:

1. The pathway from the central nervous system to an autonomic effector always consists of two neurons. One neuron leads from the CNS to a cluster of cell bodies or ganglion, in the periphery, and the other from the ganglion to the effector. These neurons may be termed preganglionic and postganglionic.

2. The ganlia of the sympathetic division lie in a chain lateral and anterior to the spinal column. Parasympathetic ganglia tend to be located near or in the effector.

3. Sympathetic preganglionic neurons have their cells bodies located in the gray matter of the thoracic and first two lumbar segments of the spinal cord[2]. The cell bodies of the preganglionic neurons of the parasympathetic division are located in the brain stem or second through fourth sacral segments of the spinal cord.

4. All preganglionic neurons, most parasympathetic postganglionic neurons, and some sympathetic postganglionic neurons release the neurotransmitter acetylcholine. Most sympathetic postganglionic neurons release the neurotransmitter norepinephrine.

Cross-Reference

Volume	Chapter
1. N1	Nervous System
2. N16	Spinal Cord

Definitions

1. Innervate: Supply with nerve impulses.
2. Effector: The target organ of a neuron.

Notes:

Autonomic Nervous System
(Parasympathetic fibers)

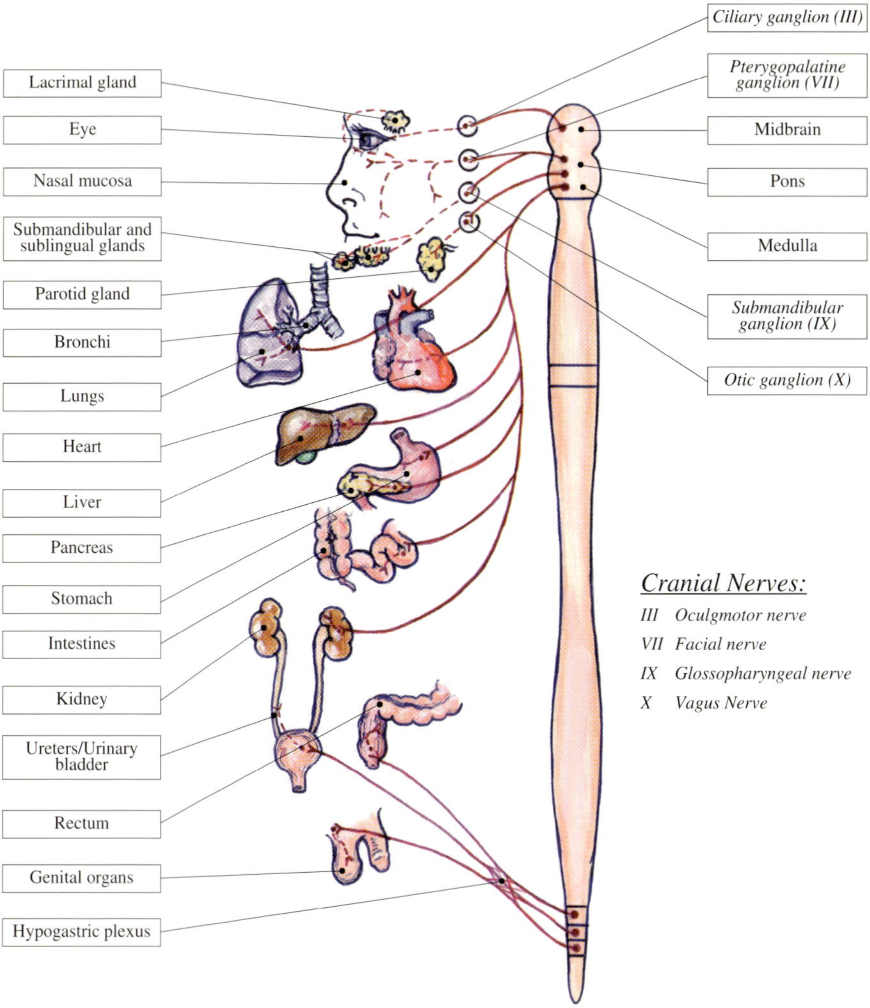

Preganglionic fibers = Solid lines

Postganglionic fibers = Broken lines

Autonomic Nervous System (Part II)

N_{18B}

III. Function:

1. The autonomic nervous system helps control the activities of smooth muscle, cardiac muscle, and many glands.

2. The effectors innervated by both sympathetic and parasympathetic divisions of the ANS are generally stimulated by one division, and inhibited by the other (dual innervation).

3. In general, sympathetic input to organs increases under conditions of perceived or actual danger (fight or flight). Parasympathetic stimulation dominates under conditions favorable for general body functioning and maintenance (rest/repose).

4. The activities of the ANS are generally not conscious and controlled by higher brain centers, notably the hypothalamus.

Cross-Reference
Volume Chapter

Definitions

Notes:

Autonomic Nervous System
(Sympathetic Fibers)

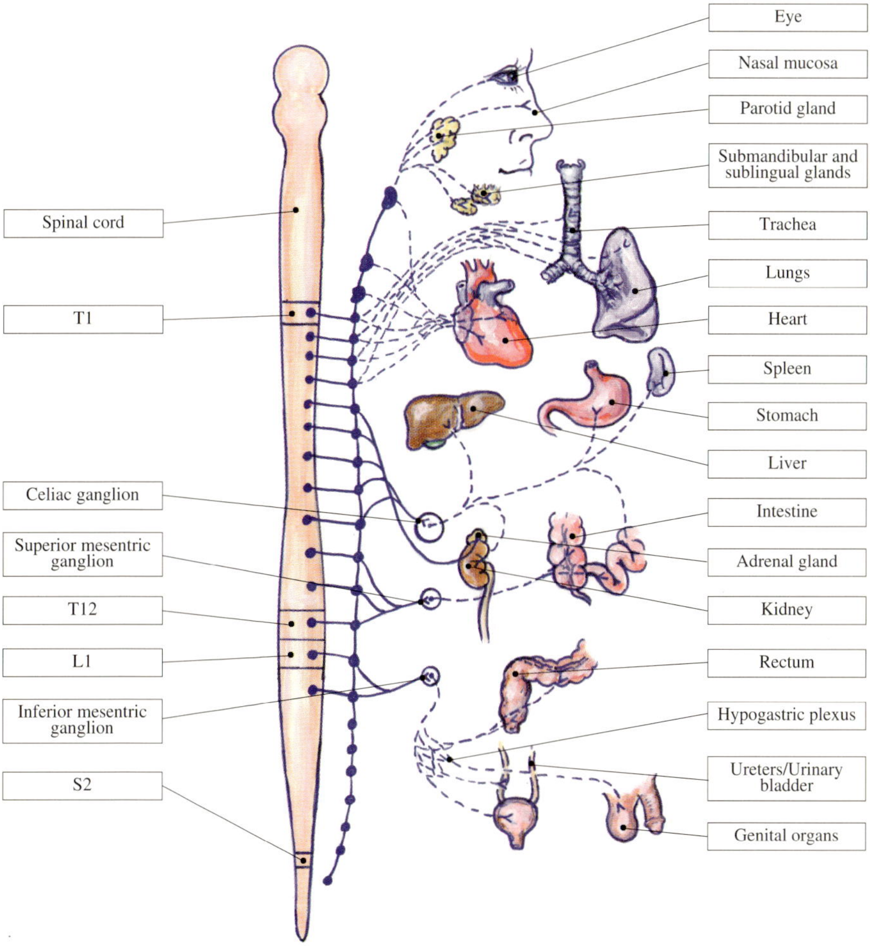

Sympathetic ganglion chain

Preganglionic fibers = Solid lines

Postganglionic fibers = Broken lines

Somatic Nervous System

N_{19}

I. Location:

1. The somatic nervous system is not a separate system, but a division of the nervous system consisting of motor neurons that innervate skeletal muscle[1].

II. Structure:

1. Where as the autonomic nervous system[2] utilizes two neurons from the central nervous system to the effector, only one neuron is involved between the CNS and skeletal muscle. Therefore, there are preganglionic or postganglionic fibers in the somatic nervous system.

2. The motor neurons of the somatic nervous system have cell bodies located in groups in the brain and anterior horns of the spinal cord gray matter[3].

3. Axons of somatic motor neurons are usually myelinated, which increases the speed of the nerve impulse[4].

4. A gap known as the neuromuscular junction exists between the end of the somatic motor neuron and the effector muscle fibers.

5. Somatic motor neurons release the neurotransmitter acetylcholine from the end of the axon into the neuromuscular junction[5].

III. Function:

1. Somatic motor neurons supply skeletal muscles with nerve impulses.

2. In skeletal muscle, acetylcholine acts as an excitatory neurotransmitter. Therefore, the somatic nervous system causes the contraction of skeletal muscle.

3. Inhibition of skeletal muscle contraction occurs only at higher centers of the nervous system, not at the neuromuscular junction.

4. Acetylcholine binds to receptors on a specialized area of the membrane around muscle fibers, the motor end-plate. This initiates a series of events in the skeletal muscle leading to muscle contraction.

Cross-Reference **Definitions**

Volume	Chapter
1. N1	Nervous System
2. N18	Autonomic Nervous System
3. N16	Spinal Cord
4. N2	Neurons
5. N5	Synaptic Transmission

Notes:

Somatic Nervous System

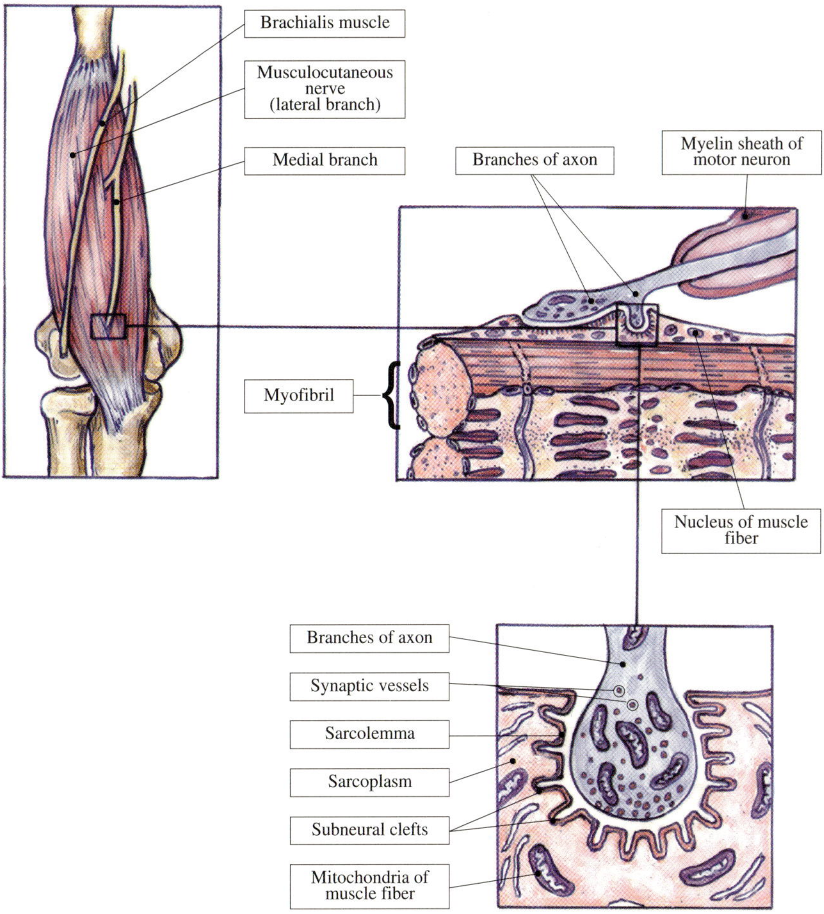

Reflex Arc

N_{20}

I. Location:

1. Reflex arcs are found throughout the body.

II. Structure:

1. A reflex arc consists of several structures:
   a. Receptor - generally a dendrite of a sensory neuron, some encapsulated in connective tissue[1].
   b. Afferent (sensory) pathway - a sensory neuron or neurons.
   c. Integrating center- the brain or spinal cord, possibly involving an interneuron[2].
   d. Efferent (motor) pathway - a motor neuron or neurons.
   e. Effector - the target organ of the motor impulse.

III. Function:

1. A receptor converts a stimulus to a nerve impulse. A stimulus may be a change in the internal or external environment of sufficient strength to initiate the nerve impulse.

2. The sensory pathway (neuron) conducts the impulse to the integrating center.

3. The brain or spinal cord (center) may initiate a responsive impulse in the motor pathway. The sensory input may also be inhibited or rerouted at the center.

4. The motor pathway (neuron) conducts the impulse to the effector.

5. If stimulated, the effector carries out a response. This may be called the reflex action.

6. Reflex actions allow the body to quickly adapt and respond to changes in the internal or external environment. These actions are generally unconscious, and provide a means for maintenance of homeostasis.

Cross-Reference

Volume	Chapter
1. I3	Receptors - Cutaneous Sensations
2. N2	Neurons

Definitions

1. Homeostasis: The maintenance of internal body conditions ideal for survival.

Notes:

Reflex Arc

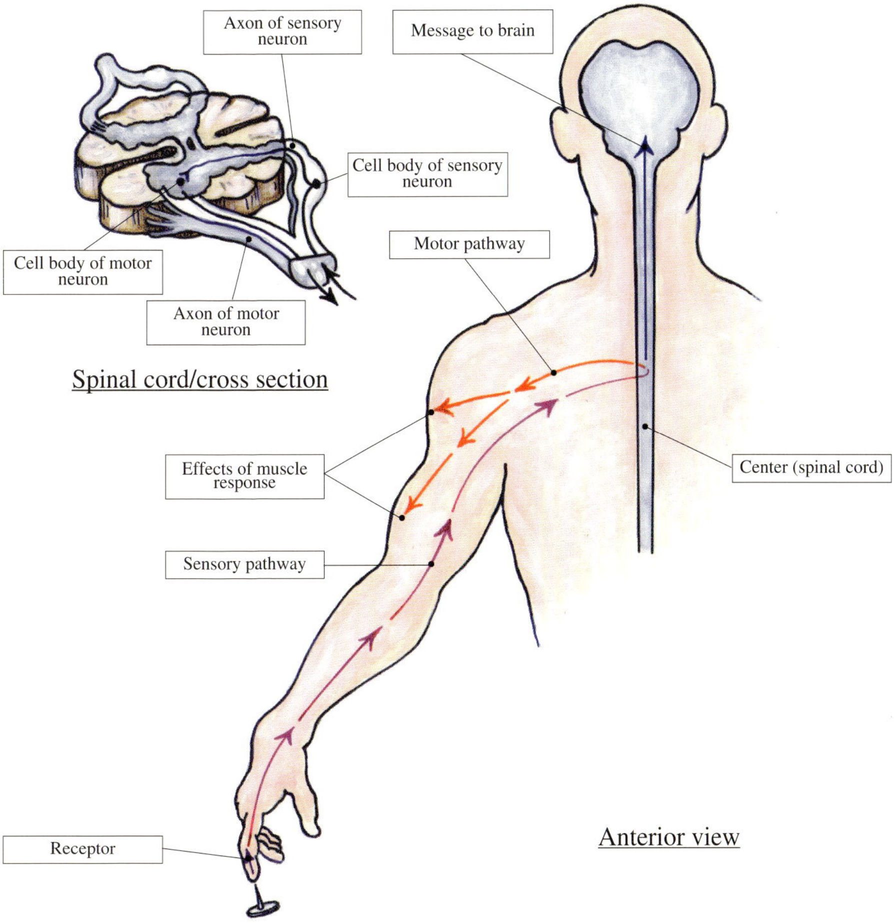

Spinal cord/cross section

Anterior view

Nervous System

Identification

(Match the letter with the term)

____ Cervical plexus

____ Radial nerve

____ Brainstem

____ Thoracic nerves

____ Ulnar nerve

____ Sciatic nerve

____ Common peroneal nerve

____ Brachial plexus

____ Sacral plexus

____ Cerebellum

____ Femoral nerve

____ Musculocutaneous nerve

____ Tibial nerve

____ Spinal cord

____ Axillary nerve

____ Lumbar plexus

____ Median nerve

____ Cerebrum

Nervous System

N_1

Peripheral Nervous System: Central Nervous System:

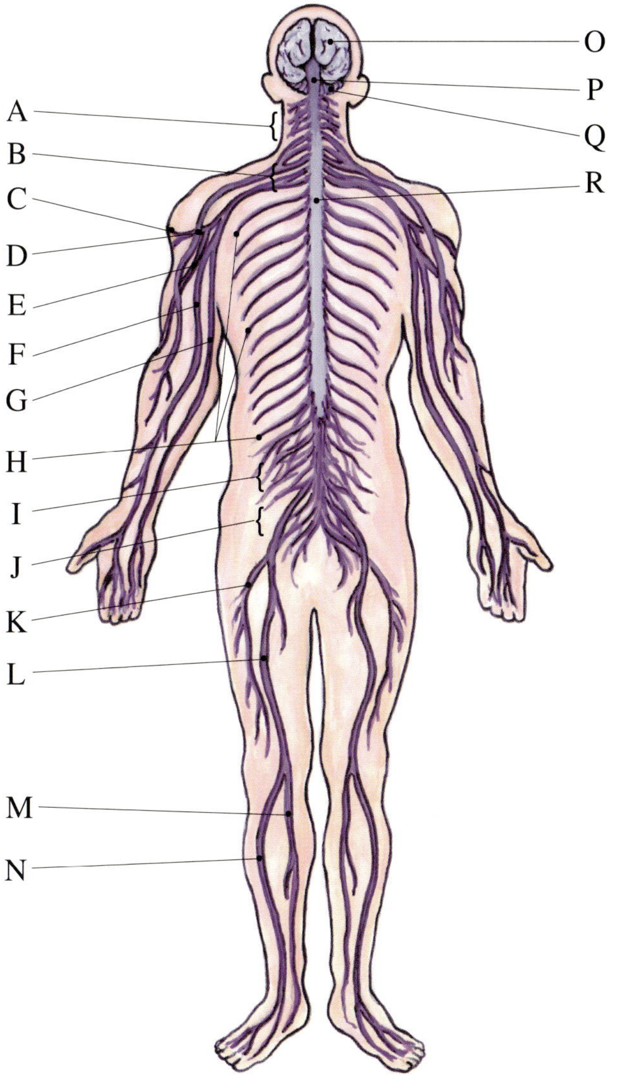

Anterior View

Neurons

Identification

(Match the letter with the term)

____ Nucleus

____ Axon terminals

____ Cell body

____ Myelin Sheath

____ Dendrites

____ Nodes of Ranvier

____ Axon

Questions

(Fill in the blank with the appropriate answer)

1. Neurons typically consist of three distinct parts:
   1)____________ 2)____________ 3)____________

2. Dendrites receive information from various receptors of the body or impulses from other ____________ and conduct impulses toward the ____________.

3. Axons conduct impulses from the cell body to other neurons or cells of a ____________.

4. Sensory neurons conduct impulses toward the ____________.

5. Association (interneurons) are located in the CNS and conduct impulses from ____________ to ____________ neurons.

Neurons

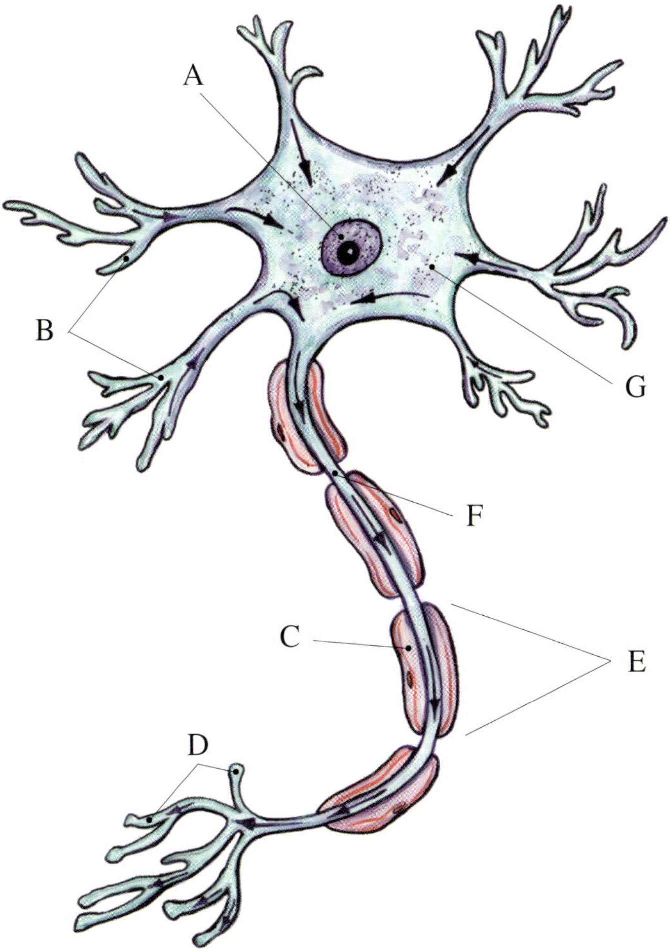

Multipolar Neuron

Glial Cells

Identification

(Match the letter with the term)

____ Microglia

____ Astocytes

____ Blood vessel

____ Astrocyte

____ Phagocytic vesicle

____ Neurons

____ Microglial cell

____ Oligodendrocytes

____ Ependymal

____ Ependymal cells

____ Process

____ Oligodendrocytes

____ Fiber of neuron

____ Microbes

Questions

(Fill in the blank with the appropriate answer)

1. Depending on shape and function, glial cells may be classified as ____________, ____________, ____________, or glial cells.

2. Astrocytes play a role in the repair of ____________ tissue, and take up excess ____________ from the fluid between the cells of the brain, preventing overexcitability.

3. Oligodendrocytes form insulating ____________ around some axons in the CNS.

4. Ependymal cells contribute to the formation of ____________.

5. ____________ are phagocytic cells from the blood that scavenge and engulf debris.

Glial Cells

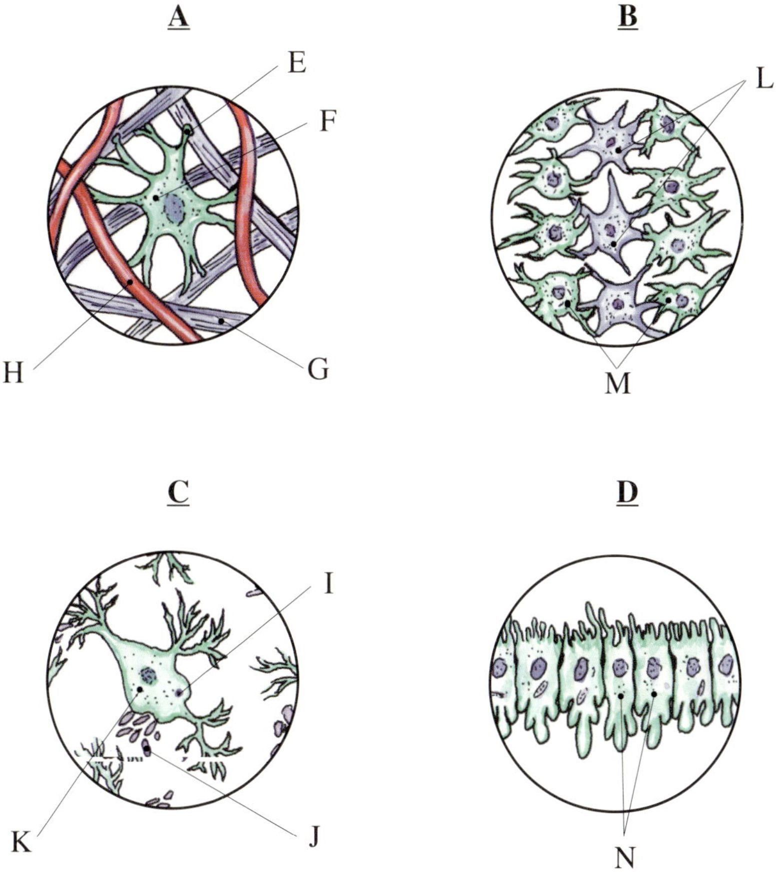

Microscopic views

Impulse Transmission

Identification

(Match the letter with the term)

____ Myelin sheath

____ Depolarized region

____ Node of Ranvier

____ Depolarized region

____ Polarized region

____ Nerve impulse

____ Plasma membrane

____ Axon

____ Polarized region

____ Depolarized region

____ Polarized region

____ Repolarized region

____ Nerve impulse

____ Polarized region

____ Repolarized region

____ Polarized region

____ Polarized region

____ Nerve impulse

____ Repolarized region

Questions

(Fill in the blank with the appropriate answer)

1. In a resting neuron, there exists an unequal distribution of ____________ on either side of the plasma membrane of the neuron.

2. A plasma membrane is said to be ____________ when the unequal distribution creates a net change difference between the inside and outside of it.

3. Unequal distribution of charges are due to the functioning of ____________ that actively transport the ions out of the cell, and ____________ that transport these ions in the cell.

4. The ____________ prevents the impulse from traveling back toward its point of origin, so neurons may only conduct impulses in one direction.

5. In ____________, depolarization need only occur in the area of the axon exposed between the insulating myelin sheath.

6. In myelinated axons the "jumping" of the action potential from gap to gap in known as ____________.

Impulse Transmission

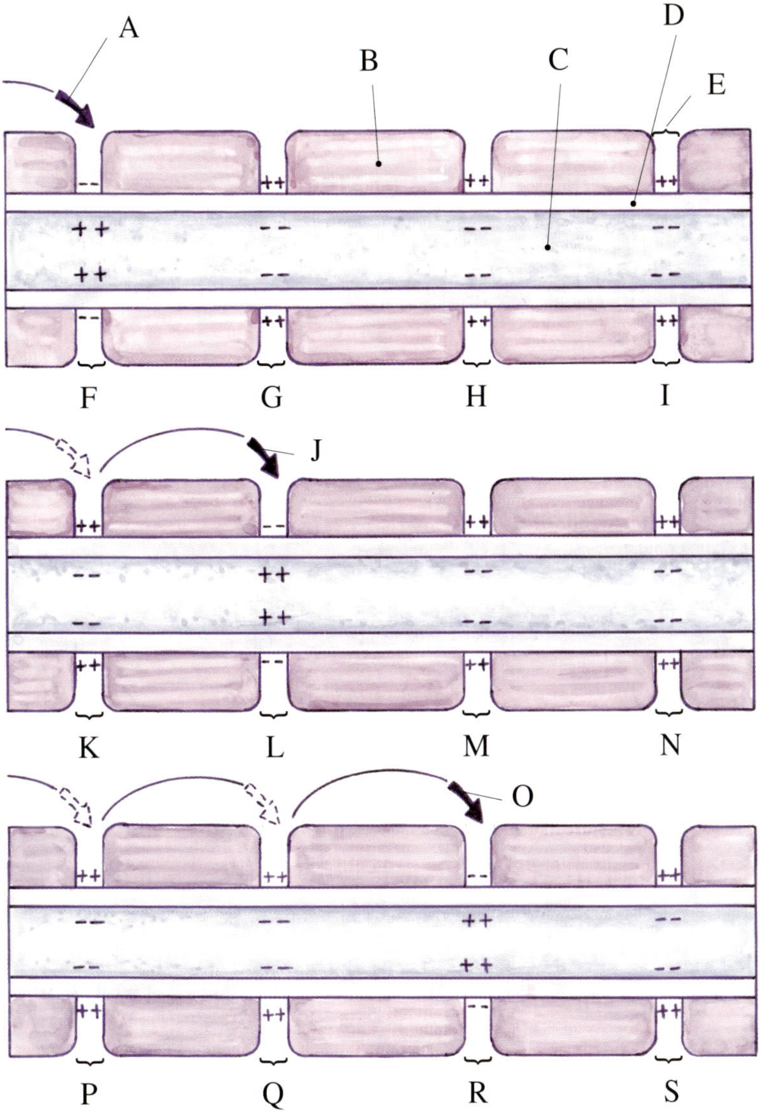

Synaptic Transmission

Identification

(Match the letter with the term)

____ Synapse

____ Synaptic vesicles

____ Presynaptic neuron

____ Presynaptic membrane

____ Release of neurotransmitters

____ Axon

____ Neurotransmitter

____ Postsynaptic membrane

____ Direction of nerve impulse

____ Nucleus

____ Postsynaptic neuron

____ Synaptic cleft

Questions

(Fill in the blank with the appropriate answer)

1. Neurons do not come into physical contact with each other, but are separated by gaps known as ____________.

2. Chemicals known as ____________ are stored in sacs in the ends of axons.

3. ____________ stimulates the release of the neurotransmitter from the presynaptic neuron.

4. ____________ effects make the postsynaptic neuron move closer to depolarization.

5. The initiation of an ____________ in a postsynaptic neuron depends on the sum of all excitory and ____________ input from presynaptic neurons.

Synaptic Transmission

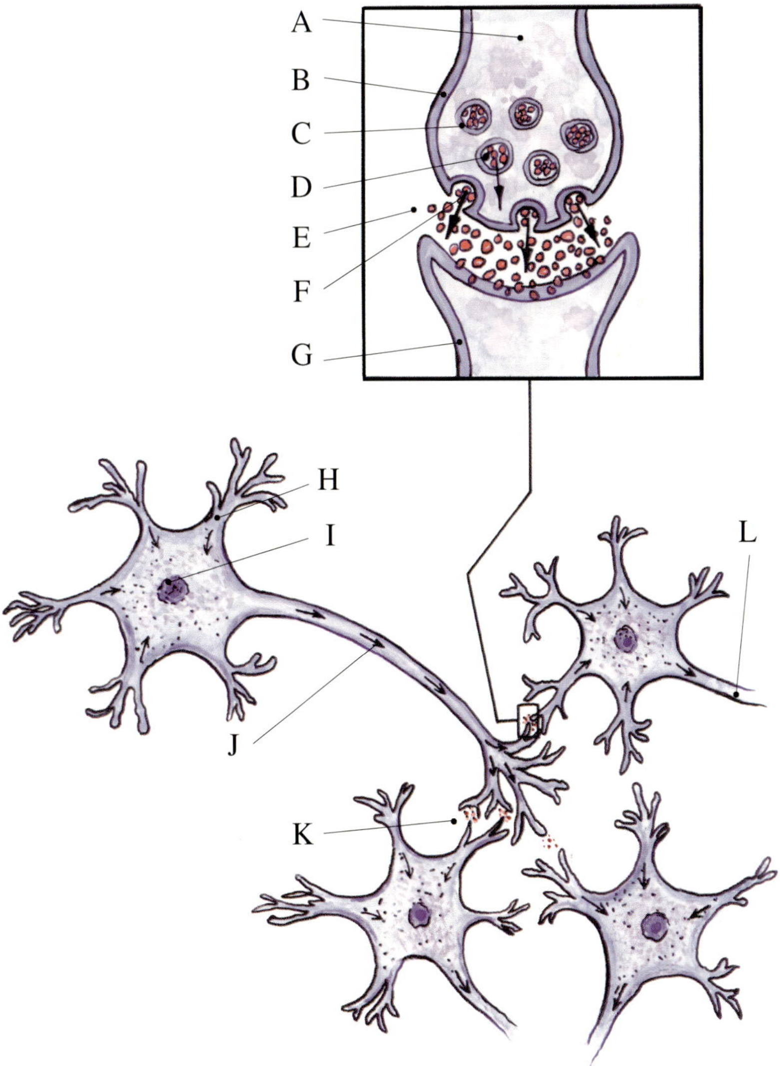

Brain

Identification

(Match the letter with the term)

____ Occipital lobe

____ Thalamus

____ Parietal lobe

____ Temporal lobe

____ Cerebellum

____ Parieto-occipital fissue

____ Midbrain

____ Central sulcus/Fissure of Rolando

____ Pituitary gland

____ Frontal lobe

____ Lateral fissue/Sylvian fissure

____ Pons

____ Medulla oblongata

____ Cerebrum

____ Hypothalamus

Questions

(Fill in the blank with the appropriate answer)

1. The brain is enclosed by the ____________ bones and ____________.
2. The brain consists of four major parts:
   1)____________ 2)____________ 3)____________ 4)____________
3. The diencephalon and cerebrum together make up the ____________.
4. The brain stem consists of the ____________, ____________, and midbrain.
5. The cerebrum includes the ____________ and ____________.
6. The brian processes input from the ____________ nervous system and ____________.
7. The brain works in concert with the ____________ to control and coordinate the activities of the body.

Brain

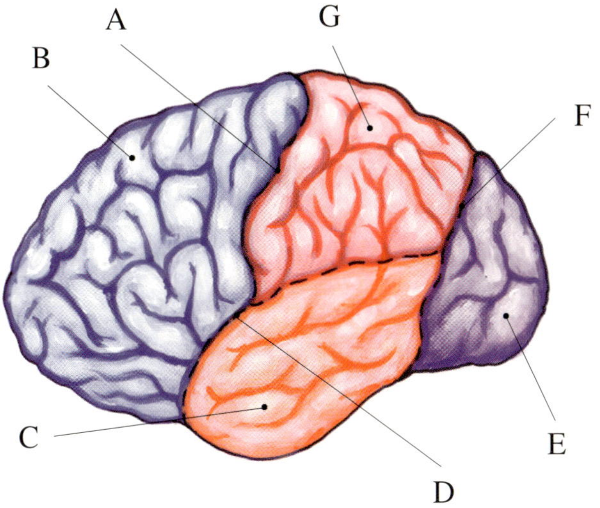

Lateral view

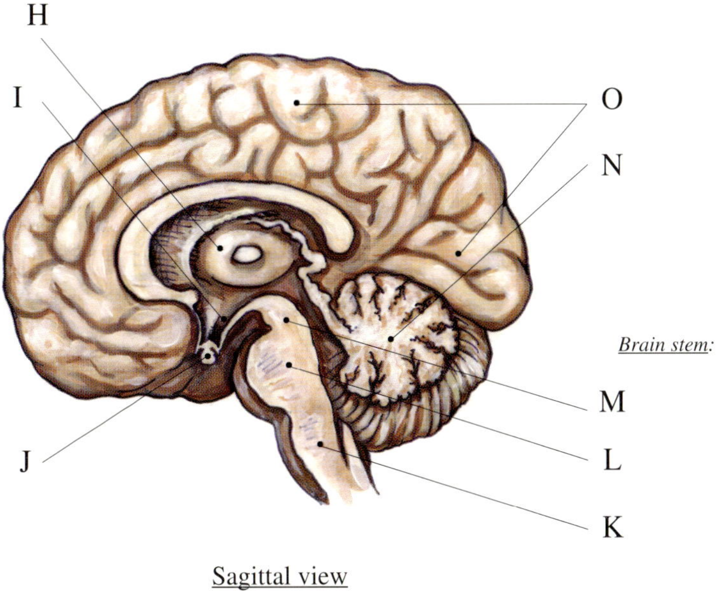

Sagittal view

Brain Coverings

Identification

(Match the letter with the term)

____ Central canal of spinal cord

____ Cranium

____ Interventricular foramen

____ Arachnoid granulations

____ Circulation of cerebrospinal fluid

____ Dura mater

____ Arachnoid

____ Pia mater

____ Superior sagittal sinus

____ Meninges

____ Subarachnoid space

Questions

(Fill in the blank with the appropriate answer)

1. The ____________ are coverings that surround both the brain and spinal cord.

2. Cerebrospinal fluid fills cavities in the brain known as ____________, the space between the arachnoid and pia mater around the brain and spinal cord and the central canal of the spinal cord.

3. Cerebrospinal fluid consists of water, proteins, ____________, ____________, ____________, and ____________.

4. The ____________ acts as a fluid-filled cushion around the brain.

5. The inner menix, the ____________, is a clear fibrous membrane that adheres to the outer surface of the brain and spinal cord.

6. Cerebrospinal fluid absorbs ____________ and circulates ____________ from the blood to the brain tissues.

7. Exchange between the ____________ feeding the brian and the CSF is highly selective.

Brain Coverings

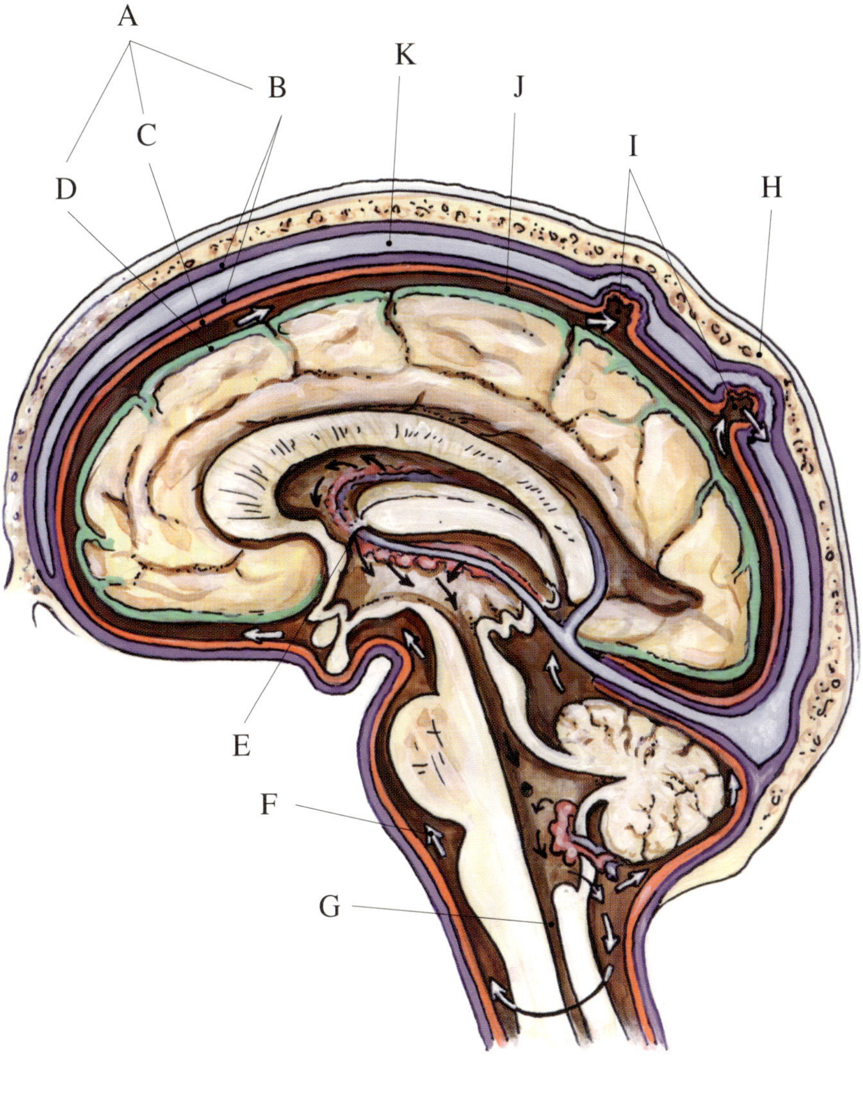

Left lateral view

Ventricles

Identification

(Match the letter with the term)

____ Suprapineal recess

____ Left lateral recess

____ Left interventricular foramen (of Monro)

____ Pineal recess

____ Right lateral ventricle

____ Left lateral ventricle

____ Third ventricle

____ Optic recess

____ Cerebral aqueduct (of Sylvius)

____ Infundibular recess

____ Median aperture

____ Central canal of spinal cord

____ Fourth ventricle

____ Interthalamic adhesion Massa intermedia

Questions

(Fill in the blank with the appropriate answer)

1. The third ventricle is connected to each lateral ventricle by a small opening, the ____________.

2. The third and fourth ventricles are connected by a small canal, the ____________.

3. The ventricles are lined by ____________, a type of glial cell, and with capillaries from the inner meninx and pia mater, these form a network called the ____________.

4. The choroid plexus from each ____________ secrete cerebrospinal fluid.

Ventricles

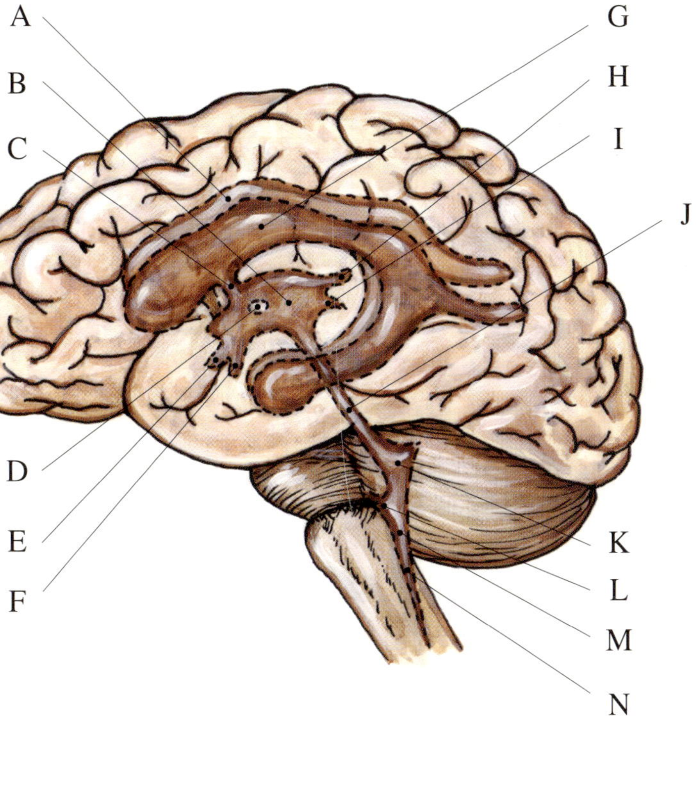

Left lateral view

Brain Stem

Identification

(Match the letter with the term)

____ Superior colliculus

____ Medial geniculate body

____ Pineal body

____ Lateral geniculate body

____ Inferior

____ Lentiform nucleus

____ Midbrain

____ Corona radiata

____ Medulla

____ Pyramid

____ Midbrain

____ Inferior colliculus

____ Olive

____ Superior

____ Pons

____ Spinal cord

____ Diencephalon

____ Medulla

____ Pons

____ Hypothalamus

____ Cerebellum

____ Middle

____ Thalamus

____ Cerebellar Reduncles

Questions

(Fill in the blank with the appropriate answer)

1. The ____________ is a continuation of the spinal cord and measures approximately 3 cm. in length.
2. The brain stem serves as a ____________ for all ascending and descending input between the spinal cord and higher brain centers.
3. The ____________ contributes to the control of respiration, sleep, and other activities as well.
4. The ____________ regulates many eye and head reflexes to different stimuli.
5. Many ____________ nerves arise from various portions of the brain stem.

Brain Stem

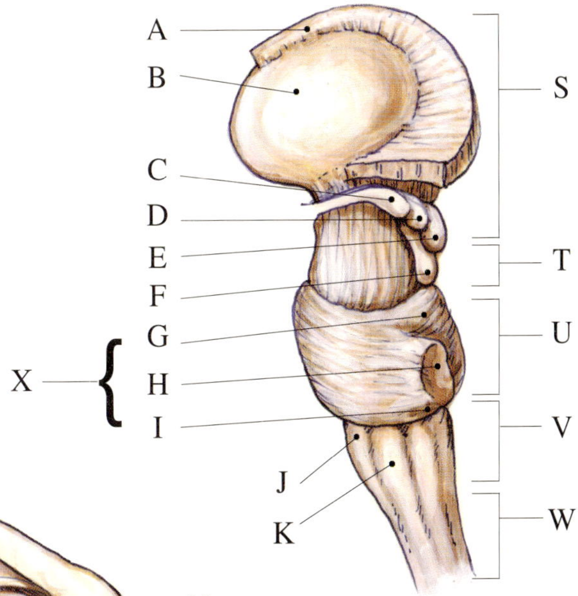

Lateral view

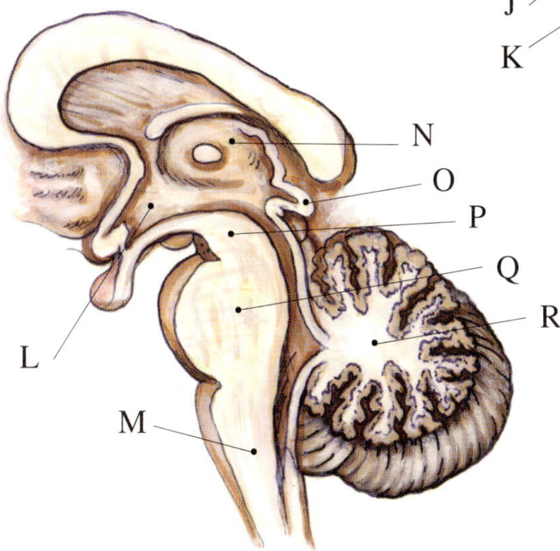

Median sagittal view

Cerebellum

Identification

(Match the letter with the term)

____ Culmen

____ Medulla

____ Tonsil of cerebellum

____ Pons

____ Cerebellum

____ Spinal cord

____ Uvula

____ Superior and inferior medullary velum

____ Tuber

____ Lingula

____ Folium

____ Declive

____ Nodulus

____ Pyramid

____ Central lobule

Questions

(Fill in the blank with the appropriate answer)

1. The cerebellum is divided into a central ____________ and ____________.

2. Bundles of fibers known as ____________ connect the cerebellum to the brain stem.

3. The cerebellum, with input from many other parts of the nervous system, maintains proper ____________ and ____________.

4. Maintenance of ____________ occurs in the cerebellum.

5. The surface of the cerebellum is corrugated by slender ridges known as ____________ or ____________.

Cerebellum

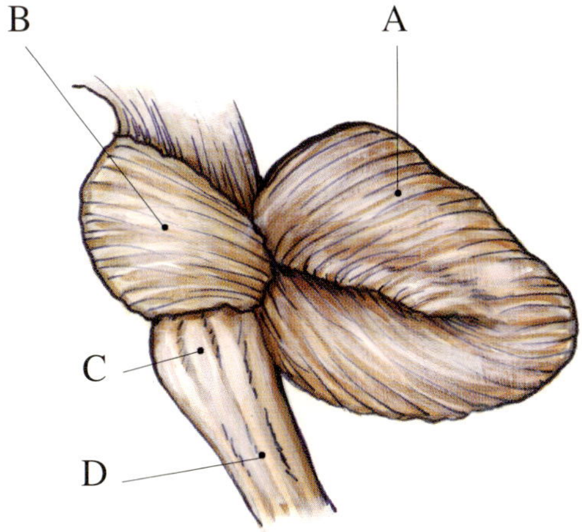

Left lateral view

Vermis of Cerebellum:

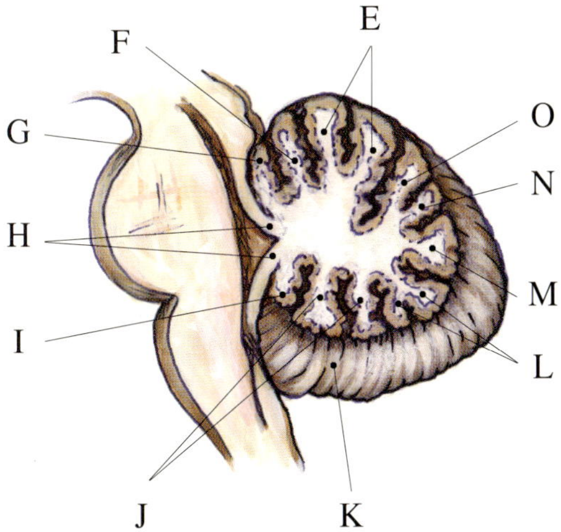

Sagittal view

Diencephalon

Identification

(Match the letter with the term)

____ Supraoptic

____ Paraventricular

____ Medial nuclei

____ Massa intermedia

____ Posterior

____ Dorsomedial

____ Thalamus

____ Pituitary gland

____ Mammillary

____ Lateral nuclei

____ Tuberal

____ Ventromedial

____ Internal medullary lamina

____ Fornix

____ Anterior nuclei

____ Lateral nuclei

____ Septum pellucidum

Questions

(Fill in the blank with the appropriate answer)

1. Each half of the diencephalon can be divided into a ____________ and ____________.

2. A stalk, the ____________, extends down the hypothalamus and connects it to the pituitary gland.

3. The thalamus screens some input, participates in a basic level of ____________ and ____________, and motor control.

4. The hypothalamus is the regulating center for many ____________ functions such as temperature, thirst, hunger, and satiety.

5. Specialized neurons in the hypothalamus produce the hormones ____________ and ____________ and secrete them into the blood through the posterior pituitary.

6. The hormone vasopressin stimulates ____________ by the kidneys.

7. The hypothalamus plays a role ____________ and many basic behavioral patterns.

Diencephalon

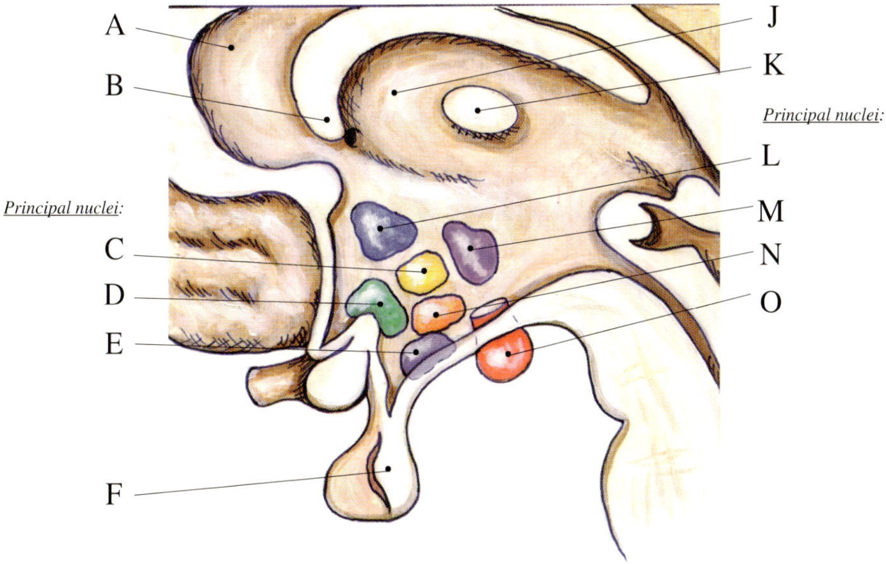

Hypothalamus: Median sagittal section

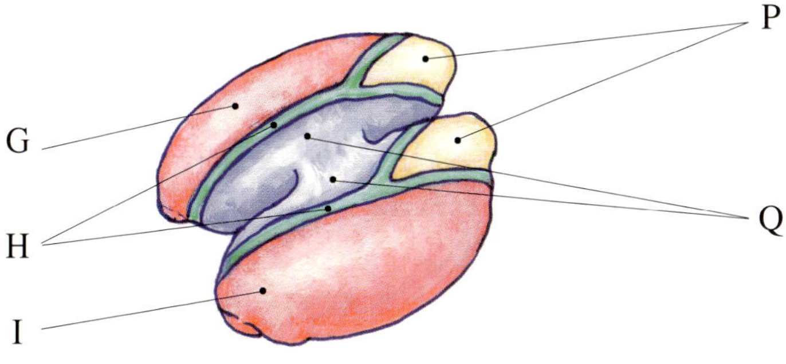

Thalamus superior/lateral view

Cerebrum

Identification

(Match the letter with the term)

____ Lacteral occipital gyri

____ Lentiform nucleus

____ Lateral fissure

____ Cerebellum

____ Argular gyrus

____ Inferior frontal sulcus and gyrus

____ White matter

____ Caudate nucleus

____ Preoccipital notch

____ Middle frontal gyrus

____ Central sulcus

____ Superior frontal gyrus and sulcus

____ Tail of caudate nucleus

____ Gray matter

____ Precentral sulcus and gyrus

____ Inferior temporal gyrus

____ Corpus collosum (genu)

_____Middle temporal sulcus and gyrus

____ Thalamus

____ Parietooccipital fissure

____ Supramarginal gyrus

____ Postcentral gyrus

____ Postcentral sulcus

____ Splenium of corpus collosum

____ Superior temporal sulcus and gyrus

Questions

(Fill in the blank with the appropriate answer)

1. The gray matter in the cerebrum is highly folded into ____________ separated by fissures or sulci.

2. The ____________ functions in most higher thought processes.

3. The ____________ generally excels at thought processes such as math, sequential problems, logical thought, and use of language.

4. The ____________ specializes in holistic or creative thought process such as music, art, or special perception.

5. The ____________ relies on its many connections to the thalamus, cerebral cortex, and brain stem to accomplish its functions.

Cerebrum

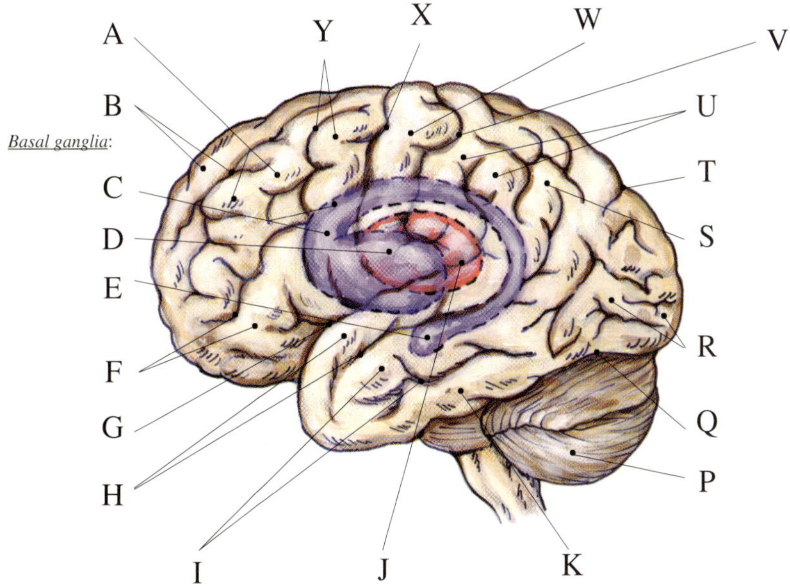

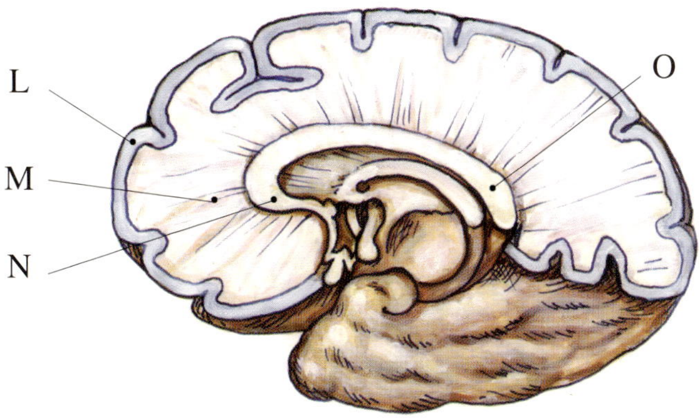

Median sagittal view

Functional Areas - Cerebral Cortex

Identification

(Match the letter with the term)

____ Primary motor area

____ Primary visual area

____ Premotor area

____ Auditory association area

____ General sensory area

____ Visual association area

____ Primary auditory area

____ Somesthetic association area

____ Frontal eye field area

____ Primary gustatory area

____ Broca's area

____ Central sulcus

Questions

(Fill in the blank with the appropriate answer)

1. Parts of the cerebral cortex do not function ____________ of other portions of the nervous system.
2. The ____________ of the cerebral cortex function in conversion of thought to speech, ability to speak, and voluntary motor control.
3. The area in the parietal lobes that processes its sensory input from the skin and related structures, is a region just behind the central sulcus known as the ____________.
4. The ____________ receive and process information about sound sensation.
5. Initial processing of visual input occurs in the ____________.
6. ____________, a region of both the parietal and temporal lobes of the left hemisphere, functions is the comprehension of verbal and written language.
7. In the left frontal lobe, ____________ plays a key role in the ability to speak.

Functional Areas - Cerebral Cortex

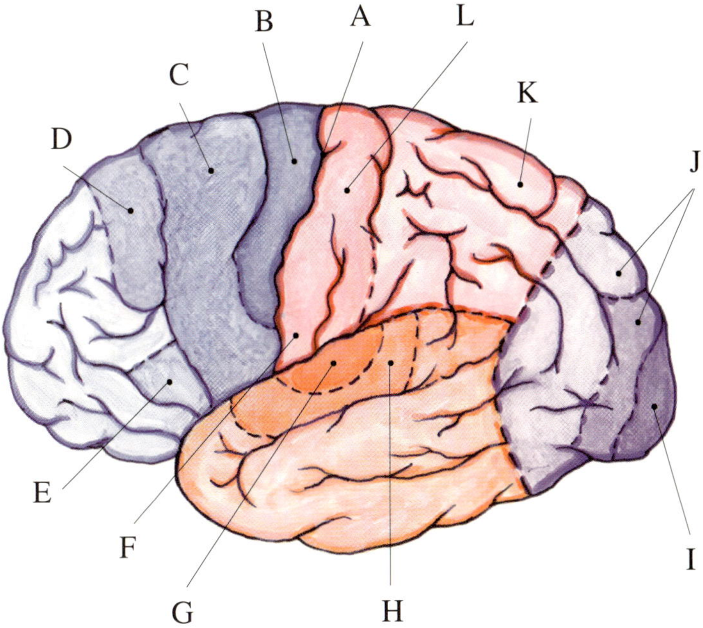

= Frontal lobe
= Parietal lobe
= Temporal lobe
= Occipitial lobe

Limbic System

Identification

(Match the letter with the term)

____ Crura of fornix

____ Commissure of fornix

____ Amygdaloid bodies

____ Body of fornix

____ Hippocampus

____ Fornix

____ Mammillary body

____ Amygdala

____ Columns of fornix

____ Cingulate gyrus

____ Mammillary body

____ Fimbria of hippocampus

____ Hippocampus

Questions

(Fill in the blank with the appropriate answer)

1. The limbic system consists of portions of several other brain parts including: ____________, ____________ of the cerebrum, and portions of the ____________.

2. Sociosexual behavior, such as ____________ is greatly influenced by the limbic system.

3. The limbic system functions in ____________ and ____________.

Limbic System

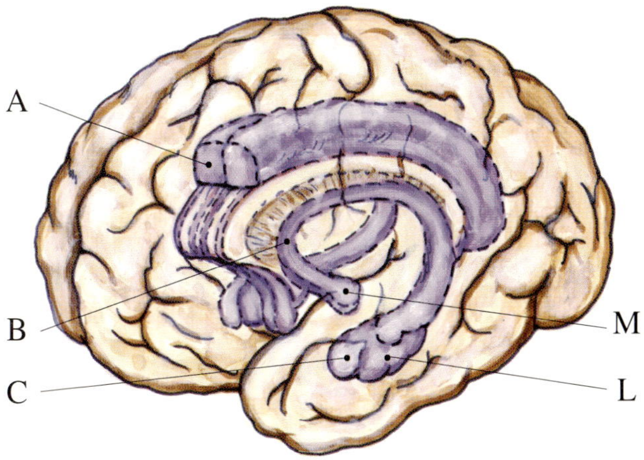

Lateral view turned slightly to the left

Fornix

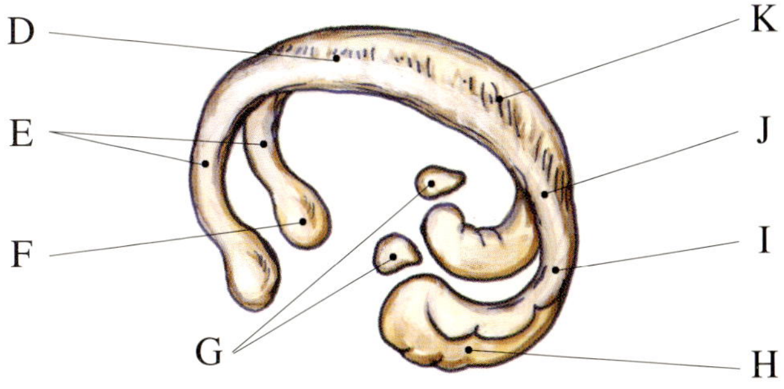

Left lateral view

Cranial Nerves

Identification

(Match the letter with the term)

____ Glossopharyngeal nerve IX

____ Hypoglossal nerve XII

____ Vestibulocochlear nerve VIII

____ Accessory nerve XI

____ Vagus nerve X

____ Abducens nerve VI

____ Trigeminal nerve V

____ Oculomotor nerve III

____ Optic nerve II

____ Trochlear nerve IV

____ Olfactory nerve I

____ Facial nerve VII (nervus intermedius)

Questions

(Fill in the blank with the appropriate answer)

1. Cranial nerves are ____________ nerves.

2. Some cranial nerves consist of ____________ only, where as some contain both kinds of neurons (mixed).

3. Cranial nerves convey ____________ to/from the brain.

Cranial Nerves

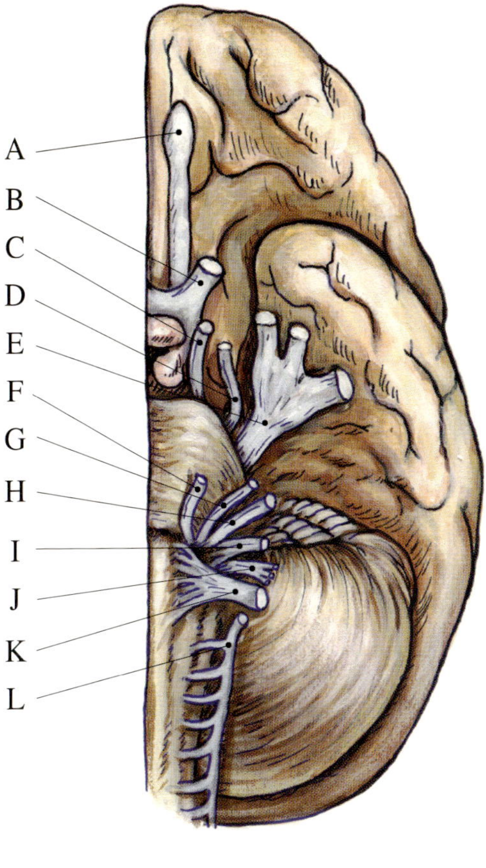

Inferior view / left cerebrum

Spinal Cord

Identification

(Match the letter with the term)

____ Posterior gray horn

____ Sympathetic ganglion

____ Lateral white column

____ Posterior root of spinal nerve

____ Spinal nerve

____ Central canal

____ Anterior gray horn

____ Lateral gray horn

____ Posterior white column

____ Spinal cord

____ Anterior root of spinal nerve/Ventral root

____ Dorsal root (sensory)

____ Anterior white coluumn

____ Autonomic nerves

____ Anterior median fissure

____ Gray matter

____ Spinal column

____ Ventral root (motor)

____ Ventral ramus of spinal nerve

____ White matter

____ Posterior root ganglion/ Dorsal root

Questions

(Fill in the blank with the appropriate answer)

1. The fibers in the white matter of the spinal cord run vertically in columns known as ____________.

2. Each spinal nerve communicates with the spinal cord by two ____________.

3. The ____________ root contains motor fibers, whereas the ____________ root contains sensory fibers, which then unite into a mixed spinal nerve.

4. ____________ tracts convey impulses from the periphery to the brain, while ____________ tracts carry motor impulses from the brain to peripheral targets.

5. The spinal cord integrates input from peripheral sensory neurons and may initiate ____________ impulses to be carried to an effector.

Spinal Cord

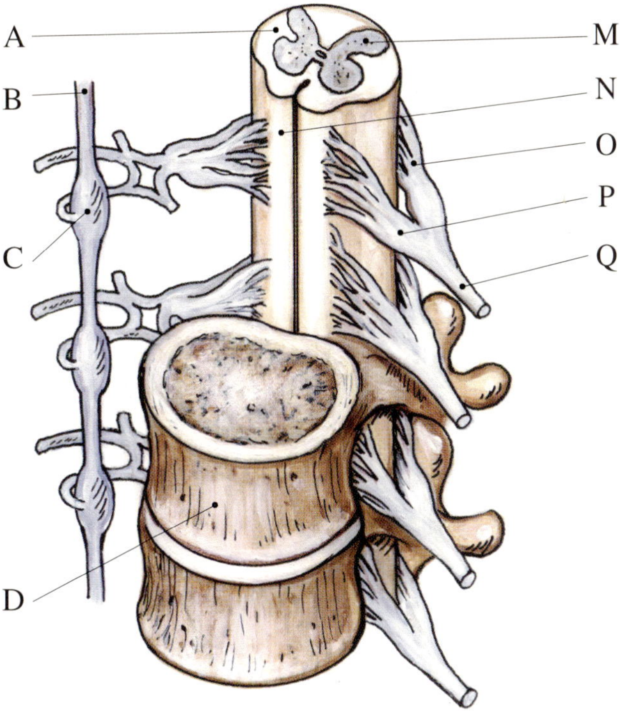

Anterior view rotated slightly to the right

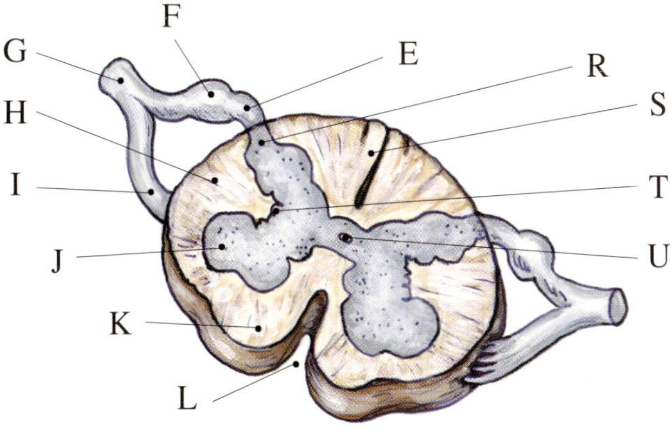

Cross-section

Spinal Nerves

Identification

(Match the letter with the term)

____ Lumbar nerves (5 pairs)

____ Musculocutaneous nerve

____ Coccygeal nerves(1 pair)

____ Cervical nerves (8pairs)

____ Lumbar enlargement

____ Sacral plexus

____ Thoracic nerves (12 pairs)

____ Ulnar nerve

____ Intercostal (Thoracic) nerves

____ Lumbar plexus

____ Cervical plexus

____ Cauda equina

____ Median nerve

____ Sacral nerves (5 pairs)

____ Brachial plexus

____ Axillary nerve

____ Cervical enlargement

____ Radial nerve

Questions

(Fill in the blank with the appropriate answer)

1. Each individual fiber in the spinal nerve is covered and bundled together by connective tissue wrappings, the ____________, ____________, and ____________.

2. Each spinal nerve branches into ____________ shortly after leaving the spinal cord.

3. Anterior rami of all spinal nerves, except T2-T12, form interbranching networks called ____________ shortly after leaving the spinal cord.

4. The ____________ plexus supplies the upper extremities, neck and shoulder regions.

5. The thoracic spinal nerves T2-T12 supply the skin and muscles of the ____________, ____________ and ____________.

6. The ____________ plexus supplies some of the lower extremity, external genitals, and abdominal.

7. The sacral plexus supplies the ____________ and ____________.

Spinal Nerves

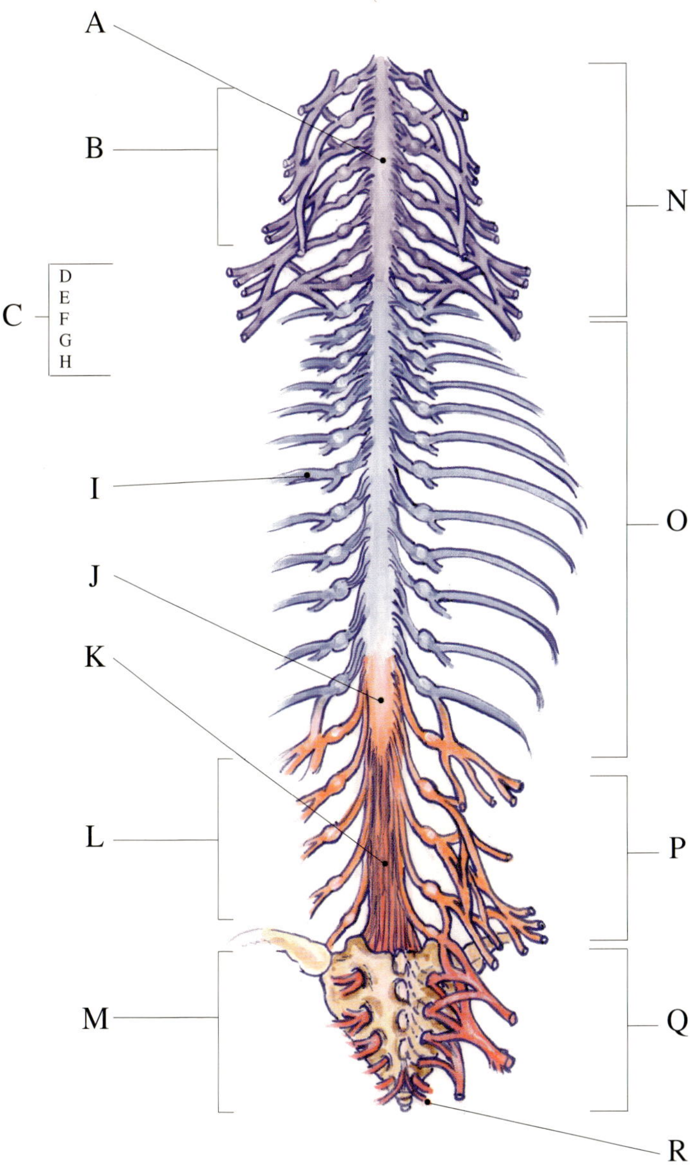

Posterior view

Autonomic Nervous System
(Parasympathetic fibers)

Identification
(Match the letter with the term)

____ Medulla

____ Intestines

____ Nasal mucosa

____ Eye

____ Rectum

____ Kidney

____ Pterygopalatine ganglion (VII)

____ Pancreas

____ Submandibular ganglion (IX)

____ Stomach

____ Heart

____ Genital organs

____ Liver

____ Midbrain

____ Otic ganglion (X)

____ Lungs

____ Pons

____ Parotid gland

____ Ureters/Urinary bladder

____ Hypogastric plexus

____ Lacrimal gland

____ Bronchi

____ Ciliary ganglion (III)

____ Submandibular and sublingual glands

Questions
(Fill in the blank with the appropriate answer)

1. The autonomic nervous system consists of motor neurons that innervate ____________, ____________, and ____________.

2. Many organs innervated by the ANS receive input from two distinct branches of the ANS, the ____________ and ____________ divisions.

3. The pathway form the central nervous system to an autonomic ____________ always consist of two neurons.

4. All preganglionic neurons, most parasympathetic postganglionic neurons, and some sympathetic postganglionic neurons release the neurotransmitter ____________.

5. Most ____________ neurons release the neurotransmitter norepinephrine.

Autonomic Nervous System
(Parasympathetic fibers)

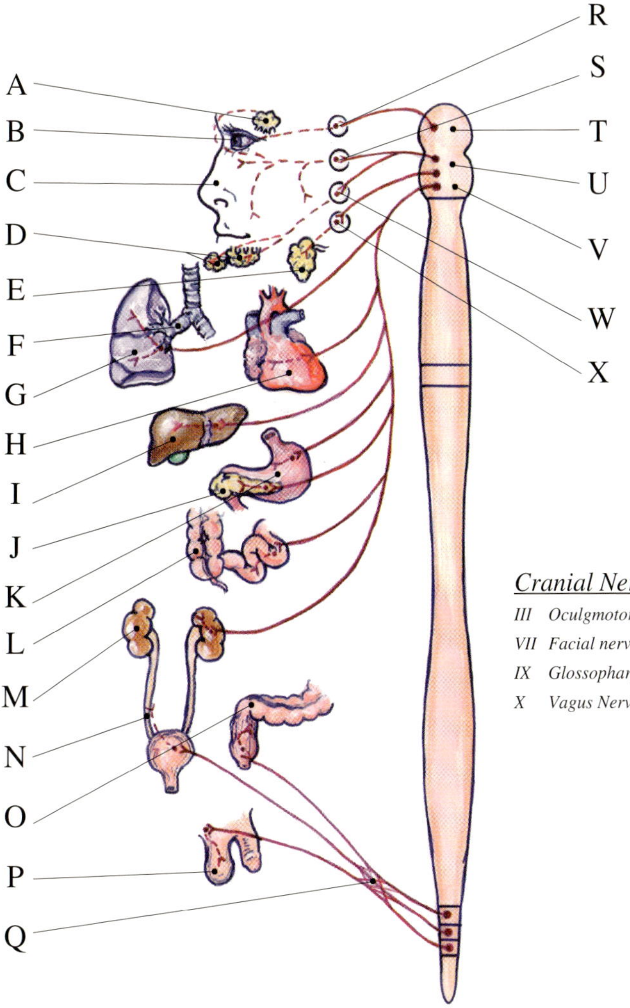

Cranial Nerves:

III Oculgmotor nerve
VII Facial nerve
IX Glossopharyngeal nerve
X Vagus Nerve

Preganglionic fibers = Solid lines
Postganglionic fibers = Broken lines

N_{18A}

Autonomic Nervous System
(Sympathetic Fibers)

Identification
(Match the letter with the term)

____ Lungs

____ Celiac ganglion

____ Parotid gland

____ Hypogastric plexus

____ Adrenal gland

____ Nasal mucosa

____ Ureters/Urinary bladder

____ Genital organs

____ Eye

____ Trachea

____ S2

____ T1

____ Submandibular and sublingual glands

____ Kidney

____ Liver

____ Rectum

____ Heart

____ Intestine

____ Spleen

____ L1

____ Spinal cord

____ T12

____ Stomach

____ Superior mesentric ganglion

____ Inferior mesentric ganglion

Questions
(Fill in the blank with the appropriate answer)

1. ____________ input to organs increases under conditions of perceived or actual danger (fight or flight).

2. ____________ stimulation dominates under conditions favorable for general body functioning and maintenance (rest/repose).

3. The activities of the ANS are generally not conscious and controlled by higher brain centers, notably the ____________.

Autonomic Nervous System
(Sympathetic Fibers)

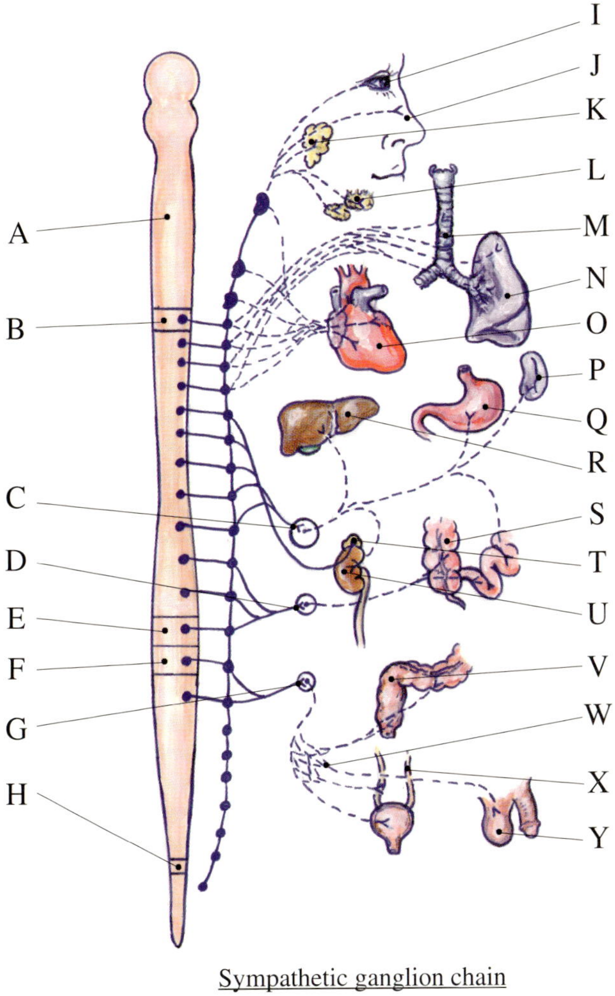

Preganglionic fibers = Solid lines

Postganglionic fibers = Broken lines

Somatic Nervous System

Identification

(Match the letter with the term)

____ Synaptic vessels

____ Brachialis muscle

____ Branches of axon

____ Medial branch

____ Mitochondria of muscle fiber

____ Myelin sheath of motor neuron

____ Musculocutaneous nerve (lateral branch)

____ Nucleus of muscle fiber

____ Subneural clefts

____ Sarcolemma

____ Myofibril

____ Branches of axon

____ Sarcoplasm

Questions

(Fill in the blank with the appropriate answer)

1. A gap known as the ____________ exists between the end of the somatic motor neuron and effector muscle fibers.

2. Somatic motor neurons release the neurotransmitter ____________.

3. In skeletal muscle, with an excitory transmitter the somatic nervous system causes the ____________ of skeletal muscle.

4. ____________ of skeletal muscle contraction occurs only at higher centers of the nervous system, not at the neuromuscular junction.

5. Acetylcholine binds to receptors on a specialized area of the membrane around muscle fibers, the ____________.

Somatic Nervous System

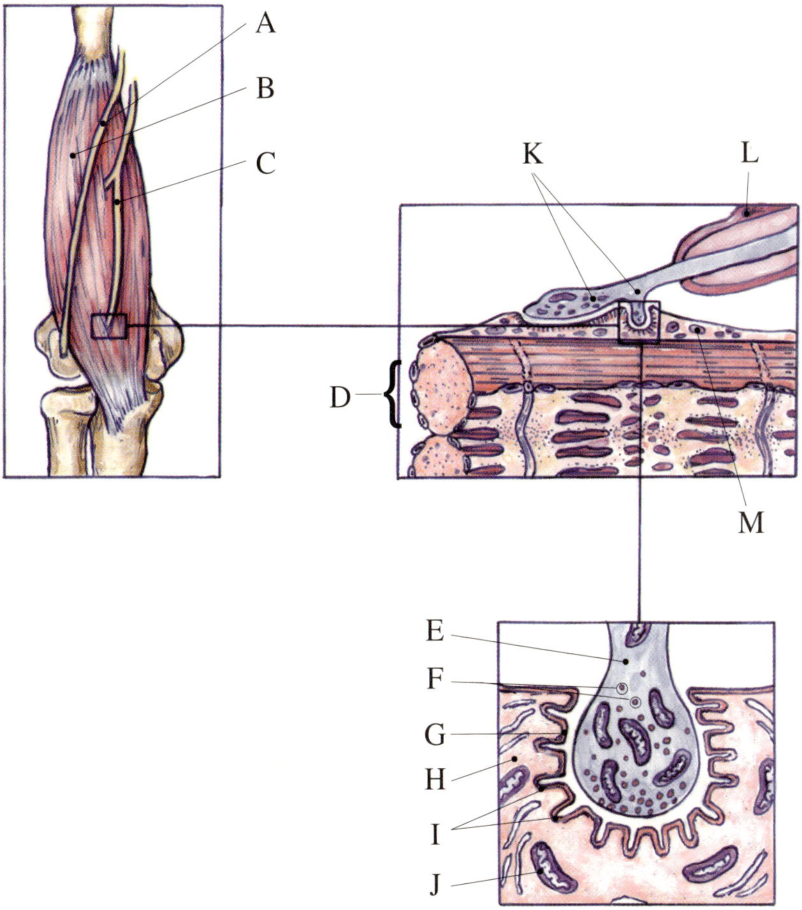

Reflex Arc

Identification

(Match the letter with the term)

____ Motor pathway

____ Cell body of motor neuron

____ Sensory pathway

____ Axon of sensory neuron

____ Cell body of sensory neuron

____ Center (spinal cord)

____ Message to brain

____ Effects of muscle response

____ Receptor

____ Axon of motor neuron

Questions

(Fill in the blank with the appropriate answer)

1. A reflex arc consists of several structures:
   1)____________ 2)____________ 3)____________
   4)____________ 5)____________

2. A ____________ converts a stimulus to a nerve impulse.

3. The sensory pathway (neuron) conducts the impulse to the ____________.

4. The motor pathway conducts the impulse to the ____________.

5. ____________ actions are generally unconscious and provide a means for maintenance of homeostasis.

Reflex Arc

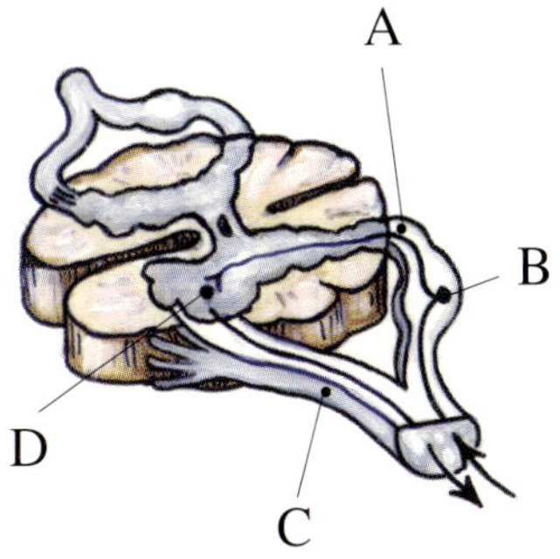

Spinal cord/cross section

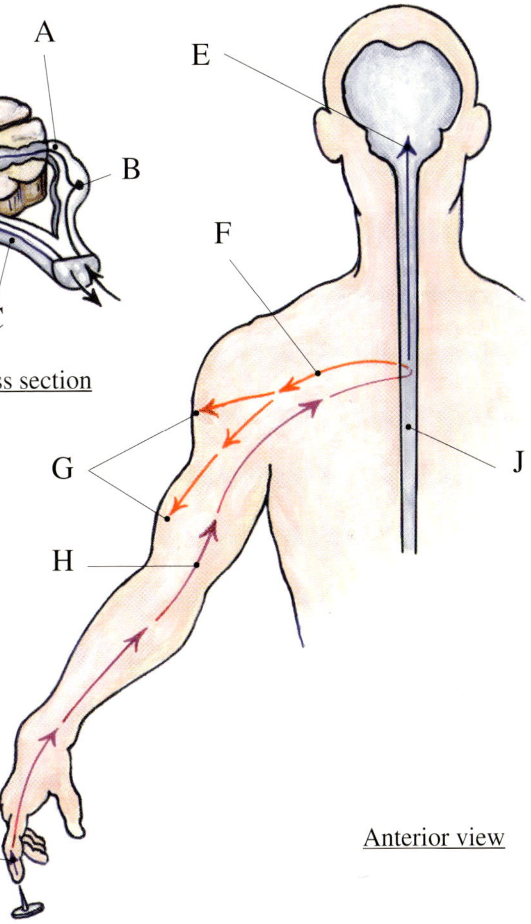

Anterior view

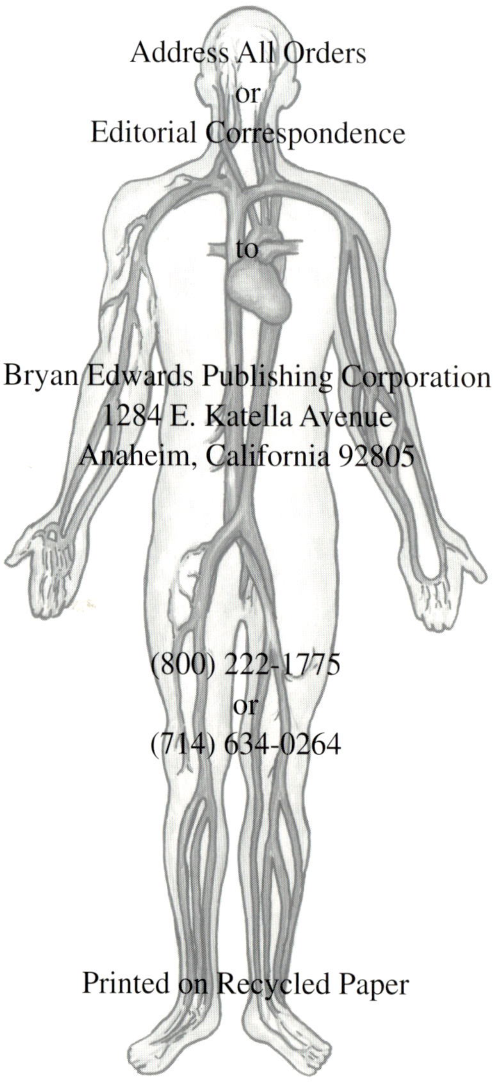

Address All Orders
or
Editorial Correspondence

to

Bryan Edwards Publishing Corporation
1284 E. Katella Avenue
Anaheim, California 92805

(800) 222-1775
or
(714) 634-0264

Printed on Recycled Paper

ISBN
1-878-576-28-3